Nurse Practitioners

Nurse Practitioners

Working for change
in primary health care nursing

Edited by Jane Salvage

Published by the King's Fund Centre
126 Albert Street
London
NW1 7NF

Tel: 071 267 6111

ISBN 0 903060 96 5

Distributed by Bailey Distribution Limited
Dept KFP
Learoyd Road
Mountfield Industrial Estate
New Romney
Kent
TN28 8XU

The King's Fund Centre is a health services development agency
which promotes improvements in health and social care. We do this
by working with people in health services, in social services, in
voluntary agencies, and with the users of their services. We
encourage people to try out new ideas, provide financial or practical
support to new developments, and enable experiences to be shared
through workshops, conferences and publications. Our aim is to
ensure that good developments in health and social care are widely
taken up.

The King's Fund Centre is a part of the
King Edward's Hospital Fund for London.

Contents

List of contributors

Nicholas Bosanquet, BA, MA, MSc, is Professor of Health Policy, Royal Holloway and Bedford New College, University of London, UK.

Tony Butterworth, MSc, PhD, RMN, RGN, RNT, DipN, is Queen's Nursing Institute Professor of Nursing, University of Manchester, UK.

John Chisholm is a general practitioner, UK.

Trevor Clay, CBE, MPhil, SRN, RMN, FRCN, was formerly General Secretary, Royal College of Nursing, UK.

Mary O'Hara Devereaux, RN, PhD, is Director, Planning and Education, Hawaii University, USA.

Marie Farrell, RN, EdD, MPH, is now Lecturer at Harvard School of Public Health, Department of Maternal and Child Health, USA, and consultant to the World Health Organization.

Ainna Fawcett-Henesy, BA, RGN, RHV, is Regional Director of Nursing, South East Thames Regional Health Authority, UK.

Elaine Fullard, MBE, RGN, RHV, DipHE, is now National Facilitation Development Officer, HEA Primary Health Care Unit, Oxford, UK.

Shirley Goodwin, BSc, RGN, NDNCert, RHV, was formerly General Secretary of the Health Visitors' Association.

Ronald King, MD, FRCP, FRCS, is now Chief Executive, Joint Centre for Educational Research and Development in Medicine, UK.

Evelyn McEwen, MA, MSc, is Divisonal Director of Services, Age Concern, UK.

Amelia Mangay Maglacas, DrPH, FRCN, ScD, was formerly Chief Scientist for Nursing, World Health Organization.

Ndiki Ngcongo, RN, PhD, is Under Secretary, Department of Health Manpower Development, Ministry of Health, Botswana.

Colin Ralph, MPhil, RGN, DN, is Registrar and Chief Executive, UK Central Council for Nursing, Midwifery and Health Visiting.

Geoffrey Rivett, FRCGP, is Senior Principal Medical Officer, Department of Health, UK.

Jane Robinson, MA, PhD, MIPM, RGN, RHV, HVT,is Professor of Nursing Studies, University of Nottingham, UK.

Barbara Robottom, MSc, BA, SRN, RSCN, QN, DNT, RNT, was formerly Professional Adviser (District Nursing), English National Board for Nursing, Midwifery and Health Visiting, UK.

Jane Salvage, BA, MSc, RGN, is Director, Nursing Developments, King's Fund Centre, UK.

Theo Schofield, MA, BM, MRCP, FRCGP, is Lecturer in General Practice, University of Oxford, and a general practitioner in Warwickshire, UK.

Barbara Stilwell, RGN, RHV, BSocSci, is a research and nursing consultant.

Barbara Stocking, BA, MSc, is Director, King's Fund Centre for Health Services Development, London, UK.

Foreword

In this era of health for all, nurses and nursing are seeking new roles that could bring about the achievement of the world's social goal of 'Health For All through Primary Health Care'. The King's Fund Centre has taken a lead in bringing together leadership nurses in education, practice (managers and practitioners) and research to review the nurse practitioner role; to explore the issues and trends surrounding the nurse practitioner's preparation and utilisation; and to seek a definitive future for her/him in health care delivery. Policy-makers, physicians, general managers and voluntary organisations also took part in the debate.

The ideas and discussions described in this report are glimpses of nurse practitioners' roles and evolutionary perspectives of them, including their effectiveness in countries with differing health systems. Some complex and perplexing issues remain. Is their practice nursing? Or are nurse practitioners filling in as substitutes in doctorless areas? Many other questions were raised and are addressed in this report, which will require further deliberation and study. Nevertheless some fresh insights and critical appraisal of the nurse practitioner's role, especially in primary health care, were stimulated. Nurses have a golden opportunity in the health for all era to create more realistic approaches to improve the delivery of health care, and the nurse practitioner concept is a big step towards this end.

This report is not a definitive text on nurse practitioners. Rather, it is an overview of ideas and a distillation of what is known about nurse practitioners in several countries. It should whet nurses' appetite to examine more carefully who nurse practitioners are and how they could shape a destiny for nursing to meet the goal of health for all. Is this wishful thinking or pious hope? I say a categorical NO! But therein lies the crux and the issue of choice – nurses can and should define their own role in the health for all era.

Amelia Mangay Maglacas
Former Chief Scientist for Nursing
WORLD HEALTH ORGANIZATION
Geneva, Switzerland

Introduction

The emergence of the nurse practitioner role in British primary health care has been one of the most exciting developments in nursing in the 1980s. It has also been one of the most controversial. What exactly is the role? Does it require special training or attributes beyond those expected of any community nurse? Is it an attempt by frustrated nurses to play at being doctors? How precisely does it benefit patients?

These questions, and many more, have been debated at length in the UK, with extra light shed on them by looking at the experiences of health care colleagues overseas. Although there is probably as yet no consensus on defining the nurse practitioner role or establishing how the needs it represents can best be met, the issues that debate raises will not go away. Far from it: the changing shape of primary and community care services in the future means they can only become more pressing.

This point is frequently highlighted in discussions in the UK following the appearance in 1987 of key government proposals for the future of care in the community. Although the papers in this volume were written before the full implications of those changes could be explored, their underlying concerns are just as topical today. Indeed they are echoed by Virginia Bottomley, Minister for Health, in an NHS Management Executive report ('Nursing in the Community', 1990). 'Those responsible for organising services', she urges, 'should create an environment in which the nursing resource is used to best effect...offering a service of the highest possible quality.'

The political climate in primary health care is therefore ripe for experimentation with nurse roles, as two British experts have recently pointed out. Nurse practitioners are at the leading edge of such experiments:

'Whatever it is called – nurse practitioner or family nurse practitioner – there is clearly a place for this role within primary care in the UK, particularly if any attempt is to be made to realise the World Health Organization's objectives of Health for All by the Year 2000' (Bowling and Stilwell, 1988).

If the nurse practitioner role is so crucial, why has no consensus on it been reached within the nursing profession, let alone agreement with other professional and managerial colleagues on the best way forward? Bowling and Stilwell hint at a major obstacle when they point out that the role is not defined solely by the range of tasks performed, nor by skill in diagnosis or treatment. 'Rather,' they say, 'the role encompasses these skills but represents too a philosophy of autonomous nursing practice, together with accountability for that practice.'

These notions of autonomy and accountability lead us straight into the quagmire of professional territorialism. Primary health care is especially swampy ground where professional boundaries are concerned because it focuses on relationships within professions as well as between them. Continuing divisions between district nurses, health visitors, practice nurses and others could mean that the nurse practitioner issue remains everybody's relative but nobody's baby.

In view of the continuing debate (and confusion) and the danger that this baby might fail to thrive, the time seemed right to gather together a group of leading nursing and medical practitioners; educators, managers and policy-makers; and consumer representatives. This might at least stimulate discussion and better understanding, and perhaps even help to map out a future path. Mutual interest in the issue brought together the King's Fund and the World Health Organization as joint organisers of the event.

The objectives of this seminar, which was held on December 1-2 1988, were to assess the need for the nurse practitioner in primary health care in the UK; to define the role; to establish whether it should be adopted and developed; to assess support for the development and spread of the role; and to recommend further areas of work. The participants were invited to attend by virtue of occupying leadership roles in nursing, medicine and health/social care, and/or because of the special expertise they could bring to bear. The complexity of the debate led to requests for a further day's meeting, which was held on May 2, 1989.

In three days of wide-ranging discussion, it was impossible and inappropriate to reach cast-iron conclusions. However, the seminar succeeded in crystallising major questions for further consideration. Clarification was thought to be needed on what work needs doing – on which issues, how, and by whom. Furthermore, it was agreed that that our starting point was not 'What should nurses do?', but rather:

- What are the needs of patients and clients?

- Who can meet those needs most effectively and economically?

- In what ways can nurses contribute?

Four particular themes emerged from the seminar discussions: developing good practices and testing innovations; disseminating ideas and experience; the preparation of practitioners; and influencing the policy process. Although there were many shades of opinion and some sharp disagreements, certain key principles underlay many of the papers presented and the statements made:

- Collaborative work is essential, including multidisciplinary/multiprofessional research and education.

- This area of practice is shaped by a variety of factors, some not readily amenable to influence from nurses, but others open to influence through a coherent change strategy.

- The maximum involvement of practitioners and service users is needed, facilitated by a supportive management environment and firm leadership at senior levels.

- Ownership of the issue is central to its successful development; in the absence of clear leadership, concerted effort is needed by the interested parties to develop strategies and carry the work forward.

Developing good practices and testing innovations

The role of the nurse practitioner, it was felt, should be developed through experimentation in the field. Rigid definition of the role is neither feasible nor desirable, but a set of underlying principles could be useful, embracing the role within the wider community as well as in relation to individual clients. There is a need to test the extent to which a new role is required; if so, who should fulfil it; what education and training is required; and how to assess its effectiveness.

Government health departments were urged to fund and encourage bids for multidisciplinary action research with a multiprofessional academic base, involving the practices of a range of professionals (in practice, education and research) in a variety of settings where good practice can be developed and tested. Quality assurance and cost-effectiveness should both be considered. These demonstration settings could include group practices of general practitioners, projects based on total health authority populations, teams of professionals working with specific client groups, and neighbourhood nursing teams.

Other demonstration projects could examine the effectiveness of models where staff have developed specific skills such as communication, decision-making, assertiveness, clinical diagnosis, community assessment and epidemiology. Undergraduate nursing courses and the impact of Project 2000 training programmes should also be considered, to evaluate their contribution to the provision of good primary health care. Finally, the part played by lay workers and informal carers – involving the community in meeting its own needs – should be considered.

Disseminating experience and ideas

Exploration of the potential of the nurse practitioner role will be most successfully tackled through a planned change programme, according to participants. This should build on an evolutionary, bottom-up approach while seizing the opportunities offered by government receptiveness to some of the key issues. Collaboration with other professions and agencies would be crucial; in particular the role needs exploring in relation to other members of the primary health care team, since there is potentially considerable overlap with the work of other professionals – although the role might enhance the work of other care providers, it might also be seen to pose a threat. The following activities should be included in this planned change programme:

- Analyse the enabling and constraining forces.

- Identify the key characteristics of the nurse practitioner role, while not allowing semantics to delay progress.

- Exploit opportunities for experiment through expanding the roles of existing staff.

- Support change agents.

- Identify a variety of models of good practice.

- Ensure effective communications to disseminate ideas – determine messages to be conveyed; ensure clarity of expression; use professional journalism and public relations skills; circulate regular bulletins; compile a directory of current good practice.

- Find ways of involving grass-roots staff and users in these initiatives.

- Identify and influence key leaders and policy makers.

- Build links with other professions, social services, voluntary organisations and others with a stake in this issue.

The different aspects of this change programme could be undertaken by various agencies, including the World Health Organization and health authorities and boards in the UK. Some participants thought that an independent, national, multidisciplinary steering group should be established to examine practice and identify good models, consider the research implications, plan developments, disseminate ideas, and draw up guidelines for flexible local interpretation.

The preparation of nurse practitioners

The need to develop skills and knowledge was highlighted, with an emphasis on drawing up appropriate training programmes – paying particular attention to the likely importance of Project 2000 in influencing community nursing, and to the Royal College of Nursing's exploration of a modular or day-release approach to NP training. Joint programmes involving both nurses and doctors could play an important role, working through bodies such as the British Postgraduate Medical Federation and the Royal College of General Practitioners.

Influencing the policy process

Developments in primary health care could be very influential in this area of professional practice; the legal implications should also be explored as soon as possible. The policy process should be influenced through a flexible approach highlighting broad development of the nursing role in general, with special reference to the Project 2000 programme, in preference to rigid definitions of roles. The key principles are protection of the public, and the establishment of practice standards.

Conclusion

The seminar raised many important and difficult issues. No clear definition of the role was agreed; as the contributions in this volume suggest, the majority of participants appeared to oppose a new, formalised division of labour in primary health care nursing. The trend rather seemed to favour continued development of all community/PHC nursing roles as the best way to meet future health care needs. The papers which follow may influence your own position on this tricky question.

Thanks are of course due to all the contributors, but also to the other participants who offered their challenges, experience and insight. Special acknowledgement should be made to Muriel Skeet, who suggested the idea; Barbara

Stocking, who encouraged me to pursue it; Amelia Mangay Maglacas, who collaborated with me so enthusiastically in organising it; Trisha Kelly, whose administrative skill and patience made this publication, as well as the seminar, possible; and Shirley Goodwin, whose support and advice was invaluable throughout.

Jane Salvage

References

Bowling, A. and Stilwell, B. (eds) (1988) *The Nurse in Family Practice: Practice nurses and nurse practitioners in primary health care*, London: Scutari Press.

Nursing in the Community. Report of the Working Group, North West Thames Regional Health Authority, December 1990.

Part I

What is a Nurse Practitioner?

The scope of practice of nurse practitioners

The first official definition of the nurse practitioner role came from the American Nurses Association in 1974. This definition was linked to statements concerning the educational needs of nurses with an expanded scope of practice. The 1975 guidelines for the Nurse Training Act, prepared in consultation with the ANA, define a nurse practitioner as a registered nurse who has successfully completed a formal program of study designed to prepare registered nurses to deliver primary health care, including the ability to:

1. *Assess the health status of individuals and families through health and medical history-taking, physical examination and defining of health and developmental problems;*

2. *Institute and provide continuity of health care to clients (patients), work with the client to ensure understanding of and compliance with the therapeutic regimen within established protocols, and recognise when to refer the client to a physician or other health care provider;*

3. *Provide instruction and counselling to individuals, families and groups in the areas of health promotion and maintenance, including involving such persons in planning for their health care; and*

4. *Work in collaboration with other health care providers and agencies to provide, and where appropriate, coordinate services to individuals and families.*

(Bliss and Cohen, 1977)

1   A global perspective

AMELIA MANGAY MAGLACAS

As the nurse practitioner appears more widely on the health care scene, people are curious to know more about the role of this emerging category of health professional in primary health care (PHC).

Nurse practitioners in PHC are professional nurses whose basic or postbasic education has given them additional knowledge, skills and attitudes, and who assume responsibility for health assessment and the management and delivery of services at the first level of a health care system.

The term 'nurse practitioner' is not so much a formal title as a form of practice and the specific training that has been designed for that practice. The titles of primary health care nurse practitioners vary from country to country; the Republic of Korea, for example, calls them community health practitioners, while in the Sudan they are known as medical assistants.

People ask, 'Why nurse practitioners?'. In 1978, countries around the world reaffirmed their commitment to the social goal of Health for All at the International Conference on Primary Health Care, and issued the Declaration of Alma-Ata, which identified primary health care as the strategy to achieve that goal. However, the success of primary health care depends on reorienting the education of all categories of health personnel to ensure that they understand the significance and intrinsic values of primary health care and are prepared to support it.

Community health nurses have long been the principal providers of essential health services to vast segments of populations, most notably in the developing countries. These nurses not only manage and staff many community health centres, they also often train and supervise community health workers and auxiliaries, and act as the first point of contact with the health care system. Moreover, nursing personnel make up the largest category of health manpower and provide a wide variety of services in many different places, including homes, schools and clinics. More than any other health professionals, they have a constant caring relationship with the people who come into contact with them.

The goal of national health services is to reach entire populations and extend the coverage of health care. The nurse practitioner provides health services complementary to those traditionally offered by doctors. This is usually cost-effective and almost always better. The nurse practitioner fills the gaps in health care that doctors were called upon to cover before, particularly among underserved groups in rural and urban communities. Interestingly, people prefer to see a nurse than a doctor when they first contact the health services. In tasks such as health assessment, counselling, and preventive health care, research has shown that nurses are more skilled than physicians.

Role and responsibilities

The role of the nurse practitioner is to carry out a wide range of primary health care services, including nursing, medical care and management, preventive care, and health promotion.

Nurse practitioners are needed in primary health care services because of their training in both prevention and cure of disease. Their responsibilities are essentially the provision of primary health care, involving them in such activities as case-finding, individual and family care, community and programme development, and health education. Other responsibilities, some of which were formerly carried out almost exclusively by doctors, include examining the sick and disabled, and treating acute conditions as well as endemic diseases. Nurse practitioners have shown themselves capable of assuming responsibility for the diagnosis and treatment of common problems and for providing continuity of care at local level. Another vital activity is the supervision and support of peripheral health workers; these are the community health workers and traditional birth attendants who give selected primary care in most of the developing countries (Mangay Maglacas, Vlin and Sheps, 1987).

While the role, functions and responsibilities of nurse practitioners inevitably vary from one country to another, as does each country's health situation, requirements, policies and strategies, they share a common response to national health priorities.

Although the nurse practitioner is generally accepted by the community and other health professionals, problems still impede their effective recruitment and utilisation. There is much work to be done on such issues as cost, acceptance, role definition and scope of practice (including regulatory mechanisms). Let us consider the role and responsibilities of nurse practitioners in different countries, including the national policies and legislation that govern their education and service.

Colombia

Colombia's nurse practitioners have since 1984 been prepared with a four-year baccalaureate programme that emphasises strongly the basic skills of nursing care, maternal and child health, nutrition, growth and development, health education, health assessment, home health and ambulatory care, research methods and management, all taught and practised in the community, as far as possible in multidisciplinary teams. Nurse practitioners assigned to clinics and health centres are responsible for the delivery of care, including screening and case management, health education, and contact with the community. They can also carry out community diagnostic studies, household surveys, and analysis of clinic records for planning and developing programmes responsive to community needs. Pending legislation will allow them a more independent role in primary health care, when the scope and limits of practice will be drawn from the content of the university degree programme. So far, though, prescription of most drugs remains outside the legal scope of practice.

Botswana

In Botswana, there was a clear policy decision to develop the primary health care nurse practitioner. A one-year postbasic course prepares them for practice in rural health centres and dispensaries where people come for comprehensive maternal and child health care and to seek treatment for illness and injury.

Jamaica

When the nurse practitioner programme of Jamaica was inaugurated in 1978, its objective was to extend basic health services to families in need of primary health care, with special attention to patients with diabetes and hypertension. The family nurse practitioner is a generalist, collecting and evaluating clinical data from health history, physical examination and diagnostic tests, and prescribing treatment to the extent allowed. They integrate health promotion and illness prevention with the treatment role, thereby addressing a broad range of health risks.

Korea and Thailand

Since 1982, the postbasic courses given in Korea and Thailand are predominantly medical in focus, preparing nurses to substitute for physicians at the level of basic health care and disease prevention.

The role of the community health practitioner in Korea is the most comprehensive and includes the management of all the most acute and chronic diseases, community assessment, home visiting, programme development and the supervision of village health workers – but only in underserved areas where no doctors are practising.

The responsibilities of Thailand's public health nurse practitioner are similar. However, little time is spent on community health activities such as assessment and planning.

Sudan

In the Sudan, candidates with a general nursing certificate and three years' experience are eligible for acceptance in the nurse practitioner (medical assistants) schools. The course enables students to acquire the knowledge, attitudes, and skills to work in a health team for disease prevention, promotion of community health, and treatment of common illnesses or conditions. The Sudanese national health plan calls for more nurse practitioners as a way to strengthen its existing health facilities and extend the coverage of health care. The nurse practitioner works under the supervision of a doctor, and as the backbone of the health services assumes the responsibility for physical examination, diagnosis, and management.

Vanuatu

In 1983 and 1984 Vanuatu trained fifteen nurse practitioners. Those working for the Department of Health were evaluated in 1988 to determine the quality of their performance in clinical, administrative and supervisory skills. They are all functioning competently, the weakest area being supervision, for which a need was expressed for further study and a practical approach for improvement.

Education and deployment issues

The experiences of these seven countries reveal both differences and similarities in the way the nurse practitioner is planned for, trained, and used. In reviewing these experiences several issues come to light. Countries need to choose the education and training options that will best prepare their nurses to assume more responsibility for primary health care. Fundamental to this is the way a country defines its nurse practitioners: an expert professional nurse who may or may not complement the doctor in the delivery of health care, or a doctor substitute, working for the most part in areas where there are no doctors. These role definitions will have a bearing on the content and length of training, whether it should embrace all the essential elements of primary health care practice or be limited to specialised functions. Countries also have to decide at which level nurse practitioner preparation should occur – at the basic level of training or at some postbasic level; in a continuing education programme or as an advanced degree.

The particular needs and social and economic circumstances of each country will be the basis for curriculum development. Training programmes have to respond to current and anticipated needs; the first efforts to expand the nurse's role in medical care through new and revised postbasic curricula came out of the pressing need to cope with health problems at community level. Now, as many common health problems such as infectious diseases and infant mortality are brought under control, there is a call for the nurse to address other essential components of primary health care, such as health promotion, disease prevention, family planning and environmental protection.

New responsibilities will require further preparation and a redefinition of the role and functions of the nurse practitioner. This, in turn, implies policy analysis and revision, and even a reassessment of regulatory mechanisms.

The legal framework for practice can either support or restrain the opportunity for broader and more extended responsibility for primary health care nursing. Although legislation governing scope of practice exists to protect the public from the dangers of inadequately trained individuals, the more specific the legislation, the more difficult it is to modify practice in order to keep up to date with biomedical knowledge and technology. The potential for restraint is also inherent in the relationship of an emergent professional group like primary health care nurse practitioners and the conservative interests of other health personnel. Even if the educational objectives of nurse practitioner training are consistent with community health needs, they will never be met if they are not congruent with the health manpower policy expressed in the regulatory mechanisms that govern practice.

While countries have introduced new approaches to training, expanding the capacity of nurses to improve both preventive and curative services to communities, where nurse practitioners work and how they function are important issues. Most countries deploy their nurse practitioners in rural areas, but if their role is largely curative, important elements of primary health care will be neglected. Although there is more primary health care nursing education, the development of service lags behind the capabilities of the nurse practitioners. Deployment and concentration in health centres and clinics, or serving as doctor substitutes, detracts from their intended purpose of providing primary care and taking responsibility for such activities as community assessment and programme evaluation.

Promoting the nurse practitioner

The nurse practitioner has become a respected member of the health team, and has for the most part won the acceptance of the community, doctors and other health workers, including nurses. Nurse practitioners have gained the confidence and approval of the people they serve because they offer increased access to curative care, health education and counselling.

While doctors appreciate the nurse practitioner's ability to assume responsibility for diagnosis and treatment of many common problems, not all accept this expanded role, even when nurse practitioners venture where doctors hesitate to tread, into isolated rural areas, for example. Other health workers (senior nurses, pharmacists, etc.) do not always understand the role of the nurse practitioner. This calls for an explanation of the nurse's scope of practice and the responsibilities that she/he is capable of assuming.

Policies may be formulated that introduce a new role into an existing health infrastructure, and legislation may be enacted to strengthen the implementation of policies. Yet unless those responsible for deployment and allocation of work have a clear understanding of the nurse practitioner's role in health care delivery, the nurse practitioner will not be best used as a key provider of health care services to the extent for which she/he has been prepared. Health planners and decision makers must ensure that this category of health professional is strengthened and institutionalised to extend health coverage effectively to underserved and unserved populations.

Reference

Mangay Maglacas, A. Ulin, P. and Sheps, C. (1987), *Health Manpower for Primary Health Care : the experience of the nurse practitioner*, Chapel Hill: University of North Carolina.

2 Nurse practitioners in North America

MARY O'HARA DEVEREAUX

A new and a deviant idea in nursing in 1965 has become one of the normative and recognised roles in nursing worldwide.

(Loretta, 1982)

The social ferment in the USA in the 1960s created crises and opportunities in all sectors, nowhere as evident as in health care. The exponential growth of science and technology after the Second World War produced a sophisticated health care delivery system and advanced levels of hospital practice for doctors and nurses, but its effects on the health of the nation were less encouraging. Access to primary care was inadequate even among the most affluent groups, and demands for improvements in primary care echoed loudly in the halls of government, industry and consumer groups. The development of the nurse practitioner must be seen in this social context.

The 1960s created an environment in which leaders seeking a change in their professions could articulate their ideas and initiate revolutionary programmes. They were helped by an increased level of social consciousness, where equity and social justice were highly valued. New programmes to improve the wellbeing of citizens could garner a greater share of resources. Such a focus on social development had not occurred since the era of President Roosevelt in the 1940s.

During the 1960s public policy on primary health care was articulated at the federal or national level, and resources were allocated to implement it with emphasis on underserved populations and cost containment. Policymakers considered these objectives essential as the American health system had become very expensive, consuming over 10 per cent of the gross national product.

In 1966, a major impetus for a new federal policy and resource allocation to Primary Health Care (PHC) was the shortage of doctors available for primary care. The development of a new concept of PHC was an important factor in the creation of the nurse practitioner. PHC was seen as a broad-based concept encompassing health and illness care. It had previously been synonymous with the general practitioner and represented a primary medical care model, but the new definition necessitated a team approach to health care and new roles for the GP and nurse. Organised medicine responded by creating the 'family physician', a new speciality to replace the general practitioner. The initiative for the development of the nurse practitioner came from both nursing and medicine.

In the late 1950s and early 1960s nursing was undergoing slow changes in education, service and research. During the 1950s nursing was more interested in hospital care and academic education; teaching and administration were given the highest status and direct patient care was considered less desirable. The 1960s saw the emergence of clinical practice and care of the underserved as more significant. Many nurse leaders feel that the role of the nurse practitioner evolved from this trend.

Concurrent with developments in nursing, organised medicine suggested that nurses should expand their roles and deliver more PHC services, under the supervision of physicians, to improve availability of and access to health care. Organised nursing rejected this suggestion as it felt that it was inappropriate, if not dangerous for nurses to take on medical tasks. The suggestion that the nurse should practise under medical supervision was also seen as a step back, since nursing had fought long and successfully to be a profession in its own right.

Academic nursing and medicine resisted the development of the nurse practitioner. The inability of nursing and medicine to communicate and plan together, and the experience with medical corps men in the armed forces gave birth to the physician assistant movement, a parallel development to the nurse practitioner (Bliss and Cohen, 1977).

Birth of the nurse practitioner

Despite the differences of opinion, a small group of nurse leaders and physicians, both in academia and in service, were teaming up to train nurses in new roles for primary health care. These leaders, motivated to improve access and availability of PHC, did not believe the tasks that doctors or nurses traditionally performed were sacred or generic to their roles. These innovators in nursing and medicine were the true midwives of the nurse practitioner; they envisaged that a new role for nursing could solve the deficit in PHC services.

Given the barriers to the development of the nurse practitioner it is remarkable that 25 years later it is firmly entrenched as a speciality of nursing. Today there are over 25,000 nurse practitioners in the USA, with about 30,000 expected in the 1990s. No other change in recent times has had such a dramatic effect on nursing.

The nurse practitioner affected health care delivery systems, educational programs, relationships with physicians and other health providers, regulatory systems that control practice, programme accreditation and certification of practitioners, and professional societies of nursing and medicine. Extensive documentation on every aspect of the nurse practitioner preparation and performance exist. No role in nursing, or in any other field for that matter, has had as thorough an investigation and description as has the role of the nurse practitioner. (Loretta, 1982)

As organised nursing witnessed the success of the nurse practitioners it began to accept them and used the movement to achieve better status for nursing in the eyes of the public and the health professions. In many parts of the USA nursing practice acts were expanded, innovations in nursing practice were created and a more functional relationship was forged between nursing serviceand education. The clinical skills of the nurse practitioner brought increased respect from doctors, although the acceptance by organised medicine diminished as the number of doctors increased and the nurse practitioner began to be seen as an economic threat.

Where are we now? During the past twenty-five years the results of the innovation have been well documented. One critical factor for the success of nurse practitioners was their contribution to increasing access to PHC and availability of services to underserved populations, particularly in rural areas. There was also an interest in the quality of their services and in their performance of medical tasks, especially diagnosis and treatment of disease. Many questioned whether patients and doctors would accept them, whether they were cost effective, and whether their education was appropriate.

A brief summary of these issues and their resolutions may provide the basis for predictions for the future in the USA and other countries (Table 1).

Table 1:   Early issues
Improve access to primary health care Increase health services for underserved Increase practice in rural and remote rural areas Be accepted by patients as a primary provider of care Provide high quality services Use new skills effectively Provide preventive and curative care Reduce the cost of care Be accepted and work collaboratively with physicians

Do nurse practitioners increase the availability and quality of PHC? As over half the patients seen by nurse practitioners are from underserved areas or populations (Sultz *et al* 1979, 1980), the answer is undoubtedly yes. Many early educational programmes were designed to train nurses from rural areas and students were recruited from areas and settings of underserved populations. This was an effective strategy for rural deployment. The ability of the nurse practitioner to increase access in rural, underserved areas may decline with the evolution of more formal educational programmes and pressure from organised nursing.

Nurse practitioner graduates from decentralised and certificate-level programmes mainly worked in underserved areas, whereas most graduates from masters degree programmes do not choose rural practice and are less likely to work in PHC settings (Cruikshank and Larkin, 1986). The US government currently provides some funding for programmes that target deployment of graduates to underserved populations, but without such support many educational institutions will find it difficult to fund innovative programmes using distance learning methods and practice based teachers. A decrease in continuing education nurse practitioner programmes will restrict the availability of PHC in rural underserved areas.

Scope of practice and quality of care

Several studies support the effectiveness and quality of care provided by nurse practitioners (see, for example, Feldman, Ventura and Crosby). One large study in a variety of settings showed a significant difference in the scope of practice of nurses and doctors, with nurse practitioners providing more educational and counselling services. Many studies describe the quality of services provided and point to the paucity of legal actions for malpractice, attesting to the NP's ability to provide comprehensive, safe and high quality services (e.g. Spitzer *et al* 1974; Runyon, 1975). Most practices of nurse practitioners are institution-based in contrast to doctors who are mainly in private practice. They occupy many positions in the public sector, thus serving the urban poor.

The nurse practitioner has created new roles for nursing in ambulatory care, making a major contribution to expanding PHC. Many service settings have created programmes around this nursing role. Although most new positions take advantage of their medical functions, their job profile has remained broad. Occupational health and mental health, health maintenance organisations and home care agencies are but a few of the areas where the practice of nurse practitioners has grown. A major determinant of the scope of their practice has been the service setting and how they define their roles in terms of the services they provide.

Collaborative practice among nurse practitioners and doctors developed in the early stages. With both nursing and medicine developing new roles, there was a need for collaborative relationships to provide comprehensive care. It is disappointing that this model has not been more pervasive, but the movement never solidified or expanded significantly – primarily because doctors perceived nurse practitioners as an economic threat.

One study reported that nurses in the team failed to adopt new attitudes to doctors. Nurses maintained the traditional hierarchical positions, with the doctor seen as the authoritative and dominant member of the team (McLain, 1988). Federal government and some states (California in particular) provided funding for the team training and practice of primary care doctors and nurse practitioners, but most nurse practitioners work in programmes where collaborative co-practice is limited. There are some interesting and successful models of co-practice in the private sector, some health maintenance organisations and family medicine residency programmes scattered throughout the USA. Unfortunately, as the traditional roles of nurses and physicians were challenged, they tended to become more competitive rather than collaborative, in an effort to retain their professional identities.

Economic effectiveness

A major concern underlying the PHC movement in the USA was the rapidly escalating cost of health care. Health care costs were driven by the costs of secondary and tertiary care. The introduction of the nurse practitioner would, it was thought, lead to significant savings although these could only be realised if nurse practitioners were part of a larger effort. In an organised system, where PHC is the entry point, GPs and nurse practitioners are the gatekeepers and case managers providing continuity of care. The combination of the family physician and family nurse practitioner, both generalist in a collaborative practice, is theoretically the best model – they can provide care to patients of all ages and sexes, particularly in rural areas where multi-specialty practices cannot be sustained easily.

The introduction of the nurse practitioner coincided with substantial changes in the organisation of services. The 1960s heralded a search for alternatives to the expensive fee-for-service, 'cost plus' reimbursement model. Health maintenance organisations, independent practice associations, preferred provider organisations and federal reforms in Medicare were all moving towards a prospective form of payment.

The economic viability of any innovation is an important concern. Could the nurse practitioner deliver enough units of care that were reimbursable in a fee-for-service system or in a prospective system to justify her salary and benefits? Were the benefits to the system sufficient to justify more nurse practitioners and fewer doctors?

The economic viability of the nurse practitioner has been demonstrated in all types of organisations (e.g. Bliss and Cohen, 1977; Mahoney, 1988; Bezjak, 1987). It is clear from such reports that they are economically feasible in a broad spectrum of PHC settings; the unsuccessful ventures have been due in large part to poor planning and a lack of information from employers. The overall success of nurse practitioners has led to support from federal and state policy for reimbursement of services delivered by nurse practitioners and acceptance of their role by insurance companies, although some of this recognition is not explicit but unofficial. The development of expedient reimbursement mechanisms has not kept pace with legislation that has expanded the role of nurses. Given that 85 per cent of the US population is covered by some type of third-party payment, explicit recognition is necessary for full utilisation of the nurse practitioner's role (Caraher, 1988). Nurse practitioners persist in their struggles to achieve this essential recognition.

Future predictions

Since the beginning of the 1980s there has been a noticeable decrease in research and evaluation of the role of the nurse practitioner, because its effectiveness and acceptance has been well demonstrated. There are areas where further research could be done to expand understanding of the role, especially in clinical outcomes, economic effectiveness and the unique contribution of their nursing background. However, these areas are difficult to research in any health organisation as other variables also influence the outcomes. It is doubtful that further findings will be a key factor in increasing the recognition of the nurse practitioner. It is up to the policy-makers, payers of care, and managers to eliminate the barriers to the full use of this resource, and to enable nurse practitioners to fulfil their potential.

The overriding issue of economics is so large in the USA that all other issues are blurred. The 1990s is predicted to be a decade of intense competition among providers. No leader in health care doubts that a national health care system based on a capitated system will be established in the early part of the twenty-first century. There will be surplus of 150,000 doctors leading to intense competition with nurse practitioners for positions perceived to be medical jobs, especially as doctors take up more salaried positions in institutional practices. The successful practice of medical functions by nurse practitioners is at the heart of the competition; if these functions are legitimised as part of nursing as well as medicine, the system will continue to use nurse practitioners, often in preference to doctors in PHC.

Where there is change and uncertainty there is also always opportunity. Leadership skills are the key to success for nurse practitioners in shaping a desperately needed new health care system for the US. There are real and unprecedented opportunities for nursing and nurse practitioners to influence the direction and structure of the system. With a clear vision they can play a leadership role: the future belongs to the visionary. In the US there is a danger that the nurse practitioner, with her genuine interest and tremendous skill in clinical care, will only focus on patient care and hope that someone else will take care of making the changes necessary to her survival – often a traditional nursing posture.

The nurse practitioner is well placed to be entrepreneurial and to form corporations which are multidisciplinary and could package services for third-party payers that are highly competitive with doctor-only services. Elderly care begs for nurse practitioners' leadership, while they are ideal professionals to serve as case managers of hospital patients. They can co-ordinate and help other professionals choose effective but least costly solutions to patients' problems. The strong clinical background of the nurse practitioner makes her a viable alternative to the doctor within her new scope of practice.

A third area of change is in quality assurance. As the USA moves to an era of limited resources, monitoring systems are required to assure quality and maintain competence. These will be demanded by all third party payers before payment.

Lessons of use to other countries

The structure and function of the American health system is different from most other countries in terms of its multiplicity of delivery models and availability of resources. To compare roles of nurse practitioners in the USA and other countries may be of interest, but the chief value of our experience may be in analysing its success and failures.

Other countries should be clear about what they are trying to change by the introduction of the nurse practitioner. Clearly, what differentiates a nurse practitioner are her advanced skills in the diagnosis and treatment of disease. She practises these skills in the context of a nursing role complemented by traditional nursing skills, and it is inadvisable to develop this role without a clear need for a nurse with these skills. There can be many uses of nurse practitioners but their development should be tied to some need in the health care system in order to use their skills or competencies effectively and efficiently. For countries with a doctor shortage, it is critical that all nurses have similiar competencies to the nurse practitioner.

The introduction of nurse practitioners was successful in the USA because considerable efforts were made by training programmes to change the legislation in order to assure the utilisation of their new skills. Working with employers and private doctors, they were able to facilitate many changes to laws, job descriptions, and supervision models. The introduction of the nurse practitioner is more than an educational programme: to be successful it demands strategic action at all levels of the system.

In countries with an abundant supply of doctors a real assessment must be made of their ability and interest in supporting or fighting the role. In the USA, the leaders of the nurse practitioner movement formed alliances with doctors and used them to assure the quality of the medical portion of the training as well as to lobby medical groups. Often nurses are too insular and unwilling to form alliances with other professionals, particularly doctors, but the ability of nurse leaders to create strategies for all levels of the system is crucial for institutionalising any significant change.

Is nursing willing to support the development of the nurse practitioner role? If so, how critical is its support? Organised nursing and most of academic nursing were actively opposed to the nurse practitioner in the USA for several years. Nursing supervisors in hospitals and outpatient clinics often showed their dislike by creating difficult working conditions for the graduates of nurse practitioner programmes. This led to requests by nurse practitioners to be part of the medical administrative division rather than nursing, arrangements which lasted for the first 10-15 years of the movement. The wounds of these early days healed slowly, and nurse practitioners and their new organisations were wary of formal relationships with organised nursing until well into the 1980s.

What are society's expectations of the nurse practitioner? If service in underserved areas or with underserved populations is expected, the selection of students for programmes and the type and level of education were the key to meeting those goals in the USA. Nurses recruited from such areas who worked there after graduation made a considerable impact on underserved populations.

Many early programmes were part of the continuing education system and not the college or university degree structure. The current trend of placing all nurse practitioner education in university-based nursing programmes and at master's degree level is reversing that trend. Organised nursing in the USA has rejected continuing education programmes because it feels they are not good for the profession, yet no other strategy has been developed to outline nursing's role in improving access and availability to PHC to the underserved.

The competency-based approach in nurse practitioner programmes developed capable clinicians. Access to adequate and well supervised clinical training has been critical in the mastery of the required skills, which often means identifying new student training sites and using doctors as faculty, at least until competent nurse faculty are developed. Linking nursing and medical faculties with collaborative training responsibilities for nursing and medical students was a step in the right direction.

The PHC nurse practitioner can have a pivotal role in twenty-first century health care in most countries. Without such a role, most developing countries have little chance of achieving the goals of Health for All. In the developed countries, some nurse practitioner skills should be part of any modern nurse's repertoire. However, considerable thought should be given to the vision that links the nurse practitioner role to improving the health status of those most in need. The vision, involvement, and persistence that leaders need to achieve the goal is considerable but the rewards are worth the effort, for both nursing and patients.

References

Bezjak, J. (1987), 'Physician-perceived incentives for association with nurse practitioners', *Nurse Practitioner*, 3.

Bliss, A. and Cohen, E. (eds 1977), *The New Health Professionals: Nurse Practitioners and Physician Assistants*, Aspen Publications.

Caraher, M. (1988), 'The importance of third-party reimbursement for nurse practitioners', *Nurse Practitioner*, 13.

Cruikshank, B. and Lakin, J. (1986), 'Professional and employment characteristics of nurse practitioners with master's and non-master's preparation', *Nurse Practitioner*, 11, 11.

Feldman, M., Ventura, M. and Crosby, F. (1987), 'Studies of nurse practitioner effectiveness', *Nursing Research*, 36, 5.

Loretta, F. (1982), 'History of a new idea and predictions for the future', in Aiken, L. (ed.), *Nursing in the 1980s: crises, opportunities, challenges*, Philadelphia: Lippincott.

Mahoney, D.(1988), 'An economic analysis of nurse practitioner role', *Nurse Practitioner*, 13, 3.

McLain, B. (1988), 'Collaborative practice: the nurse practitioner's role in its success or failure', *Nurse Practitioner*, 13, 5.

Runyon, J. (1975), 'The Memphis Chronic Disease Program: comparisons and outcomes and the nurse's extended role', *Journal of the American Medical Association*, 231, 241-44.

Sultz, H., Henry, O. and Sullivan, J. (1979), *Nurse Practitioners*, Lexington, Massachusetts: Lexington Books.

Sultz, H., Zielenzy, M., Mathews, J. and Kinyon, L. (1980), Longitudinal Study of Nurse Practitioners, Phase III, DPH Publications No. HRA 80-2, Hyattsville, Maryland.

Spitzer, W. *et al* (1974), 'The Burlington randomized trial of the nurse practitioner', *New England Journal of Medicine*, 290, 251-56.

3 Lessons learned in Botswana

NDIKI NGCONGCO

The family nurse practitioner role was perceived as essential, and formally enacted by nursing in Botswana long before formal training programmes were developed, approved and institutionalised by the Botswana Nursing Council and the Ministry of Health. To appreciate this development, we need to look at the nurse's role in Botswana, the scope of nursing practice, and the interface between nursing practice and the health care system.

The nurse in Botswana

The professional nurse in Botswana is a practitioner educated and trained to provide preventive, promotive, curative and rehabilitative services in the home, community, clinic, health centre and hospital. She carries out consultation, makes a nursing diagnosis as well as a medical diagnosis, in some remote areas initiates and prescribes investigations, treats specific conditions and refers where necessary. These interventions are seen as part and parcel of the nursing process in patient care management, whatever the setting.

In maternal and child health units, out-patient units, health centres and hospitals, almost 95 per cent of consultations and care are carried out by the nurse. Mothers coming for antenatal care, delivery, postnatal care and family planning are attended by the nurse midwife, who assesses and interviews them. About 98 per cent of mothers delivered in health facilities leave without ever being seen by a medical doctor. The nurse midwife assesses the mother in labour, monitors the progress of labour, delivers the baby, assesses the condition of both mother and child, provides appropriate care, and counsels the family on further action and home care.

All patients who enter hospitals, health centres and clinics are received by a nurse who, on the basis of her assessment, will decide whether to initiate emergency care while awaiting the arrival of a doctor. The critical judgement skills of the nurse, as well as a capacity to make informed decisions and take appropriate action, are crucial. Botswana, the size of France or Kenya but with a population of 1 million, has only 199 doctors, of whom less than 15 per cent are Botswanian. The bulk of curative, preventive, promotive and rehabilitative services are provided by nurses, of whom there are about 3,000.

The evolution of the family nurse practitioner

Nurses in Botswana informed the Ministry of Health in 1971 that while they were providing care to a variety of patients, they were not adequately prepared in physical and health assessment and consultation skills such as diagnosis, treatment and management of care. They stated that a number of their interventions were based on intuition and a limited understanding of the disease process. They did not feel they were functioning as responsible practitioners who could be held professionally accountable for their actions.

The Ministry of Health and the senior nurses agreed on the need to train nurses in consultation and management skills. This led to the development of the formal family nurse practitioner role. Six nurses were sent to the USA on a sixteen-week course which focused on maternal and child health care and family planning. They acquired some physical and health assessment skills as well as other consultation and family planning clinical skills. Back home, these nurses sensitised colleagues to the art of carrying out comprehensive physical and health assessments. They picked up abnormal heart sounds; unhealthy cervices; abdominal, pelvic and uterine tumours, and so on. They were more particular about assessing patients thoroughly before helping them to select contraceptives. Most of the nurses became aware of the importance of physical assessment skills in formulating nursing diagnosis.

In 1978 it was decided that five Botswana nurses would go to the USA for a year to train as family nurse practitioners. They were to fulfil two roles on their return: first, they would function as family nurse practitioners in five government hospitals, where they would institutionalise the role by providing an effective nursing consultation and treatment service. Second, they were to develop their hospital units as future preceptorship sites for the training of family nurse practitioners; they would also serve as preceptors and provide an internship service for newly qualified practitioners. They departed for training in 1979. A job description was developed to guide user departments in the deployment of FNPs, and meetings were held with senior nurses and doctors to clarify the concept of family nurse practice as well as the role. The FNP was described as a professional nurse practitioner who had received systematic and specialised training in the skills required for providing direct patient care, as well as preventive and promotive health services for the individual and family.

The return of the five nurses was greeted with excitement, anxiety and uncertainty on the part of nurses, doctors and other colleagues. In some hospitals, the matrons were supportive, but in a few others, they were completely overwhelmed and did not know how to handle these self-assured, clinically competent and assertive nurses, who were full of zeal and saw themselves as patient advocates. They had been trained to assess patients thoroughly and determine the tests required to check out the origins of symptoms as well as signs. They questioned doctors who made diagnoses or prescribed treatment intuitively. They demanded that patients be seen beyond their symptoms. The medical laboratories, X-ray departments and pharmacy departments felt their presence. They would ask why patients should be put on drugs such as digitalis or diuretics before obtaining a full clinical picture of their condition. They demanded specific information before they prescribed oral or injectable contraceptives. To the nurse in Botswana, the scope of practice of these practitioners was still within the parameters of nursing as practised – but the nurses who had received FNP training had a sound theoretical knowledge base. They were better prepared for providing care at home and in clinics, health centres and hospitals.

A general observation was that the more qualified, experienced and effective the doctor working with the FNP, the smoother the working relationship and stronger the team. A good example of such a relationship was observed in what was until recently our only referral hospital – Princess Marina Hospital. The doctor with his team and the FNP established a successful clinic for cardiac, hypertensive and diabetic patients which served more than 2,000 people a year. It serves as a training facility for nursing students as well as a preceptorship site for students on the FNP programme. It is a referral, follow-up, patient counselling and family health education unit.

In 1980, the National Health Institute (an interdisciplinary institution for training nurses and allied health professions) designed and developed the first FNP programme south of the Sahara with technical assistance from USAID. The development of the curriculum was a long consultative process between the National Health Institute educators, regional medical officers, district matrons, senior sisters, hospital specialists, medical doctors, the Ministry of Health, Ministry of Local Government and Lands, and private as well as mission sectors. National health policies, goals and objectives and strategies, as well as the health problems of Botswana were used as a basis for conceptualising the clinical, intellectual and other professional competencies required of the programme. Experiences from programmes in the USA and Canada were examined carefully. Literature on overseas programmes was studied in great detail.

The work experiences, strengths and gaps in performance recorded by the five FNPs trained abroad were used as a guide for designing a relevant programme. Protocols for the treatment of specific conditions were designed and developed by the FNPs, nurse educators, doctors and nurses working in remote areas. They were compared with standard treatment protocols which had been designed in the USA specially for the first few NP programmes, such as that in Kentucky developed for outreach care. Towards the end of 1981, the education committee of the National Health Institute, the Ministry of Health and the Botswana Nursing Council approved and accepted the draft curriculum, and the first fifteen students were admitted for training.

Under the technical assistance component of the Botswana/USAID Health Services Development Programme, three masters-level FNP educators initiated the programme. Nurse educators were to work as counterpart trainees and later would be trained at masters level. They would return and take over from the experts. The programme proceeded on schedule; with each new group of students, the teaching staff modified and refined their strategies and course content. The graduates provided support as they continuously assessed their knowledge, skills and performance against their work situations, and identified gaps in their knowledge and competences. Their recommendations were used as a basis for the programme review.

A survey conducted at the end of 1982 aimed to get a general feel of the practice level of the practitioners trained at the National Health Institute, the acceptance of their role by supervisors, and the availability and adequacy of support systems for their practice. It revealed that some supervisors and colleagues had not quite understood or internalised the role.

The Ministry of Health considered the following elements crucial for the successful implementation of the programme, as well as the full development of the role in Botswana:

- acceptance and understanding of the role and scope of practice of the FNP;

- acceptance and understanding of knowledge, skills and competencies of the FNP;

- team spirit and teamwork;

- effective deployment and utilisation of the FNP;

- good supervisory and management skills of nursing supervisors;

- availability of transport, supplies, equipment and medicines;

- continuous identification of the learning needs of service FNPs;

- appropriate regulatory mechanisms for guiding and supporting their practice;

- continuing education workshops, seminars and courses to update the skills of serving FNPs;

- evaluative research as well as health systems research;

- a clear career structure;

- availability of educators to continue training the cadre as well as provide continuing education;

- supportive teaching from doctors, radiographers, medical laboratory technologists, pharmacists, dentists, epidemiologists and psychiatrists;

- development of appropriate preceptor sites and preceptors;

- design and development of preceptorship tools;

- continuous dialogue between education and service;

- improvements in the design and delivery of the physical and health assessment component of the basic nursing programmes of the National Health Institute.

The Ministries of Health and Local Government and Lands and the National Health Institute had to work hard to realise these crucial requirements, and the process required much nurturing. Two strategies used for keeping track of the development were continuous dialogue with the FNPs through seminars, workshops and visits to the work sites; and reviews as well as evaluative research.

In 1985, the National Health Institute conducted a study to explore some aspects of the practice and deployment of the FNPs. The following questions guided it:

- What is the current scope of practice of the FNPs?

- How has their practice changed since the completion of the FNP postbasic course?

- How does current practice relate to their educational preparation?

- How much time do FNPs spend on the various aspects of their work?

- For what types of health problems do they most frequently provide care?

- What do FNPs identify as their successes and frustrations?

Eighty-four per cent of the FNPs said they were practising within the full scope of their practice, while the other 16 per cent felt they could be better used. Asked whether their medical colleagues were co-operative and allowed them to function effectively, 64 per cent of the respondents said they had full co-operation, freedom and support from medical colleagues; 16 per cent disagreed; 20 per cent were either working independently of doctors or hardly ever worked with them; on their perceptions of their role, 92 per cent said they were very clear, while 8 per cent gave no response. In the study sample, 8 per cent of the FNPs were in teaching positions and 1 per cent worked in a private physician's office.

It is noteworthy that only 28 per cent said some medical colleagues did not allow them to use their skills in areas such as minor surgery and management of stable hypersensitive patients. Seventy-six per cent of FNPs stated that they spent 50-95 per cent of their day on clinical consultations; 60 per cent said they hardly ever carried out home visits because they were overwhelmed with consultations. Some (32 per cent) said they spent their time co-ordinating, planning and evaluating health programmes. Three-quarters spent 5-50 per cent of their time training registered nurses, enrolled nurses and family welfare educators.

Most graduates (96 per cent) felt that their training at the National Health Institute had prepared them very well for handling medical emergencies, while 84 per cent felt that the programme had prepared them to carry out consultations and treatment fully. Most FNPs also felt that their training had increased their sense of competence; they had won the trust and confidence of the community; patients were getting better care from them; and the training had increased independence in professional practice (Pilane and Stark, 1986). These observations served as a good basis for developing continuing education programmes.

The National Health Institute also carried out an on-site survey to assess the performance/conditions of performance and solicit the ideas and perceptions of FNPs, medical officers, matrons and other nurses providing curative PHC services about improving the knowledge and skills of FNPs. This study revealed the scope and practice of FNPs as well as their caseloads. It highlighted a number of areas that required attention – placement of FNPs, conflicts with supervisors, career structure, infrastructure and other management problems (Pilane and Barton, 1986). These observations have been discussed and solutions are being worked out.

There is a lot of respect and regard for FNPs in Botswana. The public has openly recognised their worth and continues to request more practitioners for almost all our health facilities. But what is the attitude of the Ministry of Health? Top officials have emphasised their worth on different occasions. In 1985, opening the second annual workshop of FNPs, one official said:

The challenge of FNPs in Botswana is to battle for a place as an informed health provider who stands for high quality health care, to be an advocate for your patients; this means challenging your colleagues on behalf of your patients ... influencing the policy-makers to see primary health care as envisioned in the Alma Ata declaration.

The Director of Health Services, opening the fourth workshop in 1986, stated:

The FNP cadre was developed as part of the government strategy to take PHC-oriented services to the communities, and ... these FNPs serving throughout Botswana are making a vital contribution to the realisation of the goal of Health for All by the Year 2000.

And in 1988 the permanent secretary at the Ministry of Health said:

Family nurse practitioners are the most highly trained nurse clinicians in the country; and, as such, FNPs are in high demand throughout Botswana. In the clinics, health centres and out-patient departments of our hospitals, FNPs have demonstrated their competency in the diagnosis and treatment of health problems, skills which have been traditionally associated with physicians. Yet FNPs have not forgotten that they are nurses, and they have combined these new curative skills with the 'caring' which has traditionally characterised the nursing profession.

To date we have a total of eighty FNPs assigned to hospitals, health centres, clinics and educational institutions. The following questions come to mind:

• Has the development of the FNP cadre weakened or strengthened the traditional role of the multi-purpose registered nurse in Botswana?

• Are FNPs regarded as physician assistants or independent, interdependent professional practitioners?

• How can Botswana ensure that when nurses enter further studies to improve their clinical and management skills, they are admitted into programmes that will truly build on their consultation and direct patient care competencies?

- Can Botswana ensure that the FNP skills in family and community health, as well as in public health practice, are as strong as their patient care clinical intervention skills?

- What is the contribution of FNPs to nursing knowledge?

- Is the programme impacting on other nursing education programmes?

- Is the programme an expansion of the basic four-year nursing programme, or is it a postbasic nursing specialist programme?

The programme graduates are only just beginning to consolidate their role and to expand their scope of practice. They are carrying out research; one is involved in research on AIDS, some are looking at patient satisfaction with the services they provide, and others are looking at deployment and career mobility patterns of FNPs. We have identified the following areas for strengthening the training programme: material and child health and family planning technology, cancer screening, occupational health, research, health education, family health care and management.

We believe this innovation has made some difference to the quality of service provided by nurses in Botswana. The challenge is to strengthen the basic nursing education programme, to avoid spending too much of the postbasic training of FNPs on reinforcing anatomy and physiology, chemistry, microbiology and social sciences which had been poorly taught or insufficiently covered during the first four years of nurse training.

The FNP should not be bogged down with simple tasks which a registered nurse midwife can deal with. The government must seek ways of improving the working conditions of nurses in Botswana and demonstrate a recognition of nursing specialist skills as they do for medical specialists; otherwise the health care system may not sustain the current motivation levels of FNPs. They will have to be considered for leadership position in areas of direct patient care. Their continuing education needs must be carefully analysed to ensure that the programmes developed for them are academically and professionally sound. The educators of FNPs should be clinically competent practitioners in their own right.

Botswana plans to support the programme at any cost.

References

Ministry of Finance and Development Planning (1980), *National Development Plan V 1980-85*, Gaborone: Government Printer.

Ministry of Finance and Development Planning (1985), *National Development Plan 1985-91*, Gaborone: Government Printer.

Ministry of Health (1986), *Revised Curriculum for Training for Family Nurse Practitioners Post-Basic Course*, National Health Institute, Gaborone: Government Printer.

Pilane, C. and Stark, R. (1986), 'Botswana family nurse practitioners as primary health care providers; an evaluation study', *Botswana National Health Bulletin*, 2, 3, 391-402.

Pilane, C. and Barton, T. (1986), Report of the on-site observational survey of the practising family nurse practitioners in Botswana. Unpublished.

4   A European perspective

MARIE FARRELL

While many parts of the world still ponder over the elusive notion of health for all by the year 2000, the WHO European Region has set itself an agenda with a specific mandate. The mandate is to address and achieve the thirty-eight health targets set by its thirty-two member countries between now and the turn of the century. The implications for innovative approaches to nursing and care practices are enormous: and the possibility of a nurse practitioner nursing practice is attractive and, in some places, very sorely needed.

In Europe, the countries talking about these ideas and other ideas often associated with nurse practitioner activities are the UK and Sweden.   Most of the development, research and evaluation has been done in the UK. The research is in its infancy as is the practice, but positive evidence has been documented concerning patient outcomes, patient satisfaction, cost issues, health team members' responses and the effects on nursing involvement in prevention. The extent to which the time spent on prevention actually alters illness patterns is a subject under study for other kinds of practitioners as well.

It is well known that physicians who are paid on a salary basis will spend more time in health promotion and disease prevention than those paid on a fee-for-service basis. As most nurse practitioners are salaried, one might ask: is it the practitioner role that is the variable of interest, or is it perhaps the way the person is paid that accounts for the difference in emphasis on prevention or treatment?

Considerable discussion continues on the nurse practitioner's skills to improve the quality of health care versus his/her ability to provide cheaper first-contact care than that provided by physicians. In the European literature, most studies underscore the physician's helper role and the time and labour of the physician that is saved. With more time available some physicians complain that they have little to do, yet they do not tend to use this time to deal with health promotion and disease prevention. This seems to bear out the views of those who say that even if they have the opportunity and time, doctors will not deal effectively with the caring elements of practice. Yet the thirty-eight European health targets, for the most part, do not deal with mortality or morbidity. They focus on client functioning, client choice and issues of cost – the raison d'etre of the nurse practitioner.

These developments in nursing are in keeping with several other trends which have taken place over the past fifty years.

Today's issues – yesterday's solutions

Let us look at three ideas. The first has to do with your great grandmother and you. When your great grandmother lived, married and raised her family, life was tenuous, hard and short. She died at 55 or 58 and had many children, some of whom themselves died in childbirth. Families had lots of illnesses, many with no cures, and many meant crises and life/death situations. For you, the story is different. You may live well into your late 80s, have two or three careers and one or two children (maybe at home or at a birthing centre). In all probability, the births will be normal, or uneventful, as we say in the business. Life is not one life-threatening crisis after another, and we don't have seven or eight children in order to be sure one or two of the toughest survive.

Your family's pattern reflects the changes in health eras. At the beginning we had infectious diseases (polio, tuberculosis, malaria); after they had been dealt with we faced not acute but chronic long term conditions (mental retardation, cancer, heart disease). You may not die of cancer, you learn to live with it. Finally, we have the lifestyle era of alcohol and drug abuse, unemployment, family breakdown, and one new horror which covers all three eras – AIDS.

From this brief profile, we can see that what our grandparents dealt with was profoundly different from what we face today. Yet we are trying to address today's issues with yesterday's solutions. We do not need as many people educated to save lives or to treat infectious diseases. Hospitals all over the developed world are closing units and consolidating; people in hospital are there because they are very ill and need twenty-four hour nursing care, and are often discharged much earlier than they would have been even ten years ago. Let us take the example of AIDS and the projections for the future. By 1990, half of the hospital beds in New York will be used for people with AIDS, at a cost of $50,000 per person. Putting people in hospital because no one is home to care for them or because families need a weekend off or are burned out from twenty-four hour care are some of the challenges we face. We need carers, providers, volunteers – communities with very different ways of providing support. In short, we are educating health providers for cure when we need care, for acute situations when actually they are more long term, and for the single solution when the drug problem will take multiple solutions. Our universal imperatives for care go beyond mortality and morbidity. The focus is on everyday functioning and client choice.

Three periods of time can be identified that mark major changes in the ways the health sector has formed their objectives, functions and capabilities: the individual care era, the community care era and the population care era.

Individual care era

During this era (up to the Second World War) the curative care of the individual was the dominant theme. The number of patients who could be cared for was limited by the capacity of the providers able to render services.

This pattern persists today in many parts of the world. Available money is spent supporting speciality areas, often those that are glamorous, high tech and intellectually stimulating to the providers. Thus, it is very common in poor countries to see literally scores of providers in hospitals in the capital and rural areas with virtually no health care available.

The community care era

The community care era (from the Second World War) was the time when attention was given to health services for larger portions of the populations, and to increasing the emphasis on public health and prevention programmes. During this time, services went to particular groups, such as the pre-schoolers, or to a special element of primary health care, such as nutrition. A two-tier system developed where the health professionals provided care at the hospital level and auxiliaries provided care in health centres or dispensaries.

The research/educational institutions continued to be focused on cure, and a biomedical model of care prevailed. Many had progressive views of public health and health care, but the schools of public health were not highly influential in either their universities or their countries in shaping health policies and directions. Health care and services were provided for or to communities. Your mother was told by Dr Spock how to raise you, and Carl Rogers helped hundreds to congruence with no more than an 'uh-huh' during the 50-minute hour. WHO provided advice, not collaboration. We were the experts, the people were the recipients of our knowledge.

The population care era

The population care (Health for All) era focuses on universal coverage, with primary health care as the key concept. Universal coverage is developed for a defined population. In this present era, the password is access. The debate in the UK is a HFA issue. Should a person have access to a health centre if he/she cannot pay? Why are there people here who want universal coverage or national health insurance? What's wrong with a system based on private practice? This same debate rages in North America, but with the opposite questions raised. Why are there people who want a national health system? What's wrong with their competitive system?

There is plenty wrong with all of the present systems. For one thing, most countries are producing the wrong types of personnel for the wrong kinds of care for often the healthiest groups. Although twenty-five out of thirty-three European countries in one report showed that 100 per cent of their populations had access to PHC, the number of people available to provide those services is quite small.

Seven countries reported a range from 11.54 nurses to 100,000 population, to 157.6 nurses per 100,000. The number of midwives for six countries for PHC ranged from 1.3 to 31.2 per 100 000 population. The number of physicians for eight countries ranged higher, from 39.38 to 77 per 100,000 population. According to Abel-Smith, 'there can be no rational defence of a situation in which there is one doctor to three or four nurses in several northern European countries and one doctor to 1.5 nurses in southern-eastern Europe' (Abel-Smith, 1986). These figures must be viewed cautiously, however, because international studies on health professions are extremely rare. Not all countries collect equivalent data and conceptual difficulties exist in defining, even approximately, the limits of each profession studied.

Having made these rational observations, some other factors must be considered. Like all other actions which can be perceived as homing in on another discipline's territory, the nurse practitioner movement may be seen as being in competition rather than in collaboration with other professionals. Even though the service may be cheaper, as effective, and more relevant to the needs of the population during the HFA era, and even if the skills performed are of no interest to another provider group, the nurse practitioner may not be welcome. From experiences here and in other parts of the world, it is clear that the factors which affect his/her acceptance depend on the perceived need, the way the practitioner introduces and presents him/herself and the needs of those whose practice may be the most affected. Where the other providers are mature, comfortable with their skills and professional body of knowledge and have positive past experiences with members of a health team, the chances for positive outcomes are probably enhanced.

If the nurse practitioner is seen as one more in a series of attempts to reduce, change or interfere with others' practices, especially where there is an excess of providers to begin with, the chances of acceptance by some other team members may be reduced. However, this does not mean that the efforts should not go forward. We all know that what is good for a provider may not be what is necessary for successful client outcomes. If the health targets are the focus in this lifestyle population care era, the needs of the client or patient are the concern. Society has put the professional responsibility on health providers to ensure effective, efficient services. That is the nature of the professional beast. It is up to us to decide how best to fulfil that mandate: that is the challenge for Europe for the future.

Reference

Abel-Smith, B. (1986), 'The price of unbalanced health manpower', In Z. Barkowski and T. Fulop (eds), *Health Manpower Out of Balance: Conflicts and prospects*, Mexico: CIOMS.

5   The British scene

AINNA FAWCETT-HENESY

The last two decades have witnessed a virtual revolution in the ways in which individuals, families and populations wish to direct their own lives. Nowhere is this trend more evident than in their wish to take control of their own health and sickness: note the public, informed debate about the future of the British National Health Service, the role of the doctor, and the place of preventive care, as well as the success of particular groups (notably women) in challenging professional behaviour. Others have cleverly influenced government policy (such as mentally ill people), or harnessed charitable and voluntary power to augment their choices in health care (such as elderly people).

What has caused such a shift in expectation, in expression of need? In some ways the development of medicine during the last 200 years could be seen as an aberration; these changes may merely be a return to the norm. For most of human history the management of sickness, health, childbirth, child development, old age and death has been a matter for individuals, families and communities, with practitioners seen to be interacting with natural forces. The biomechanical rationale for modern health care, which arises from a Cartesian view of the world, is beginning to be questioned. It is becoming apparent that the mechanistic approach has largely failed to improve health; furthermore it is seen as dogmatic and restrictive.

In the UK and much of Northern Europe, health care is mostly directed towards repair of individual and isolated disorder, which until recently has not been seen as either an individual or a social responsibility. But it is now time to return to people-directed health and sickness care, to environmental and ecological approaches, to healthy lives, and to open, easy access to care.

A good litmus test of whether a service is satisfying requirements, or even needs, is whether alternative services are filling gaps in the market. The development of the role of the nurse practitioner is generally seen to arise from inadequacies in the provision of medical care. This has been the case in the UK, the USA, Scandinavia, and parts of the Third World. In the UK the development has occurred for three main reasons:

- A lack of appropriately qualified and experienced medical practitioners, e.g. in accident and emergency departments (Barking, Havering and Brentwood Health Authority 1988).

- Patients' dissatisfaction with the quality of care – including consultation time and choice of available treatments, as in primary health care (Stilwell, Greenfield, Drury and Hull, 1987).

- Difficulties in access to primary health care (Burke-Masters 1986).

These problems are well demonstrated in comprehensive studies of the provision of British health care. The 1942 Beveridge report and the ensuing 1946 NHS Act were formulated on the proposition that providing socialised sickness care would gradually reduce the population's need for services. More recently, the Black report (Townsend and Davidson, 1982) identified large sections of the population which were receiving no health care at all, or were receiving a discriminatory and therefore inadequate service. In 1988, The Nation's Health (Smith and Jacobson) asserted that most people lacked opportunities to prevent their own ill-health, were excluded from preventive services, and possessed little knowledge about how to acquire the information they needed.

Evidence of this nature indicates that medical resources are inadequate; it also directs attention towards resource usage and efficiency. These two factors, more than any other, have probably determined the emergence of alternative forms of care provision.

The provision of state funding has led to date to a conservative and controlled health service. Alternative, imaginative provision is almost always independently funded and/or unregulated; neither is satisfactory. In the present culture of consumer participation, informed decisions, individual choice, and demand for high quality and flexibility, the professions have a duty to respond and nurses must play a full part.

The role of the nurse practitioner in the UK has therefore developed in areas where resources are under scrutiny; where patients are able to express and have expressed dissatisfaction; where they can be offered choice – albeit limited – and where they are not generally so ill as to be unable to make that choice; and, perhaps most importantly in terms of further role development, where the nurse can be the primary point of access for patients. The role itself has developed in two ways:

- As a member of a highly skilled primary health care team.

- As a known specialist in the care of a specific client group, e.g. children, women, or homeless people.

British nurse practitioners have generally developed the first aspect of the role in two areas: general practice surgeries and accident and emergency departments.

General practice

In this model the patients have open access to the nurse practitioner. In Stilwell's study (1987), a total of 858 patients of all ages and ethnic origins sought consultations for 979 problems. Morbidity from every diagnostic group was presented but 60 per cent fell into the 'supplementary' group: preventive medicine, health instruction and education; social, marital and family problems; and administrative procedures. It was felt that most patients chose a consultation with a nurse practitioner appropriately, and in more than a third of consultations the nurse managed the presenting problem without further referral for investigations, prescriptions or medical advice.

The nurse practitioner in the second model works alongside the general practitioner; both are equally available to the same patient population over the same period. In one scheme the nurse practitioner saw a similar age and sex distribution of patients to the doctor but saw different types of problems. More of her patients needed follow-up of chronic diseases, health advice and screening measures, while fewer were acutely ill. The doctor dealt with four times as many patients. The nurse practitioner managed 78 per cent of her consultations without referral to a doctor, and 89 per cent without resorting to prescribed drugs. Patients were very satisfied with her work and 97 per cent of those who saw her would choose to consult her again.

Accident departments in general hospitals

In one project in this setting the nurse practitioner was a registered nurse with over five years' accident and emergency experience. She acted as an alternative professional as a first point of contact for those visiting the department with minor ailments. The outcome of the project was increased satisfaction for patients because of reduced waiting time, and a reduction in the numbers seen by the doctor. It appeared that patients appreciated the advice and reassurance they received from the nurse practitioner. Her practice was also deemed safe.

In the USA and Canada, the second role predominates. The nurse practitioner has developed as a doctor substitute rather than as an alternative practitioner. Care of children, the elderly, and chronic diseases are the most common specialist areas associated with the role. However, family nurse practitioners have been developed in Canada, and work is ongoing at McGill University in developing the nursing component rather than the medical component of the role.

Whatever the model or setting, seven characteristics appear to be important:

- Direct/primary access.

- Choice for patients.

- Diagnostic and prescribing powers for practitioners.

- Authority for referral.

- More personal attention during the consultation.

- Time.

- Counselling and health education.

The development of nurse practitioner roles has emerged in isolation from wider policy issues. At the same time there is a paucity of evaluative research, in the UK and elsewhere. Why does the nurse practitioner appear to achieve better outcomes than the doctor? While we know much about how nurses interact with patients, we know very little about what affects the final outcome. We also need to look at ways of categorising patients other than by medical diagnosis, in order to find out what nurse practitioners are contributing in social terms. Research is also needed on which patients are willing to use a nurse practitioner and why. The effects of education and experience on the nurse practitioner's practice needs to be investigated, with a view to finding those nurses best suited to this work.

In summary, although the roles developed by nurse practitioners across the western world have been diverse, their characteristics are similar. Whether these characteristics account for the known outcomes (improved patient compliance, increased trust and confidence, more patient satisfaction) is as yet unresearched and unresolved. However, several features of their practice receive repeated mention and merit further study.

The development of the nurse practitioner in the UK has been slow and restricted. In both the accident department and general practice, it has taken place under the auspices of the medical profession, and owes much to shortfalls in the services provided by doctors. Under such circumstances the public may expect nurses to replace doctors. Consumer surveys about the sort of service they desire demonstrate concerns with availability, access and length of consultation – matters other than the presenting condition.

References

Barking, Havering and Brentwood Health Authority (1988), *The role of the nurse practitioner in accident and emergency services at Oldchurch Hospital, Romford.*

Burke-Masters, B. (1986), 'The automonous nurse practitioner – an answer to the chronic problem of primary care', *Lancet*, 31 March, 1266.

Smith, A. and Jacobson, B. (eds) (1988), *The Nation's Health: A Strategy for the 1990s*, London: King Edward's Hospital Fund for London.

Stilwell, B., Greenfield, S., Dinny, M. and Hull, F. (1987), 'A nurse practitioner in general practice: working styles and pattern of consultants', *Journal of The Royal College of General Practitioners*, 37, 154-57.

Townsend, P. and Davidson, N. (1982), *Inequalities in Health: The Black Report*, Harmondsworth: Penguin.

Part II

Are Nurse Practitioners Needed?

6 Setting our professional house in order

TONY BUTTERWORTH

My starting point for this paper is a belief that patient and nurse are bound together in a symbiotic relationship. There are those who might argue that idealised models have no place in real life, but I believe in at least aiming for an ideal type.

Why people want nurse practitioners in the first place and what their expectations of them might be is a matter of some debate. Indeed, the central question must be who most wants to see the development of nurse practitioners: nurses, consumers or government? All have something to contribute towards developing the role, evidence shows stronger support from some of these groups than from others.

Pioneering work by nurses and health visitors at an individual practitioner level is well represented by the work of Burke-Masters and Stilwell. These individualistic efforts made a significant contribution to developing the role of the nurse practitioner; however, to develop this role across the whole profession opens a new chapter of development for nursing in the UK. Individual effort can be safely categorised as 'experimental', 'unique', 'eccentric' or 'meeting the demands of a local need'. It is more contentious to advance on a wider front as the consequences are far-reaching, affecting intra-professional nursing relationships, inter-professional relationships, and most importantly of all, nurse-patient relationships.

Collectively, nurses in the UK have a strong professional voice in the Royal College of Nursing. Their stance is clear and two recent RCN documents, Boundaries of Nursing and Specialities in Nursing (1988), make the case for developing elements of the nurse practitioner role.

The first document suggests that:

the boundaries of nursing must be able to respond to
people's needs. Educational curricula and official
guidelines, however, tend to change relatively slowly.
It is nurses themselves who are faced with making
the decisions as to what they will, and will not do, since
each nurse is accountable for his or her professional
practice. Clearly there is room for professional growth
within these boundaries.

The second publication makes the case with greater
force: 'If the profession of nursing is to reach its ultimate
goal of providing relevant nursing care to meet individual
patients' needs, then ultimately the role of the nurse
specialist is central to its achievement. This claim builds
on propositions that nurse specialists are experts in a
particular aspect of nursing care – 'they demonstrate
refined clinical practice, either as a result of significant
experience or advanced expertise, or a knowledge in a
branch or speciality'.

These identified areas are clearly critical for a
developing nurse practitioner role, and the profession has
staked a claim which determines two steps leading to a
nurse practitioner grade – expert knowledge or clinical
skill, and permission to break the boundaries of previously
defined roles. This popular rise in professional
development can also be seen in a collective response to
papers from government (1986) which have sought to
address contentious issues such as prescribing by nurses
and evolution of a nurse practitioner role in primary care
(the Cumberlege report and the primary health care
discussion document). The RCN's response to the
consultation on primary health care initiated by the UK
government health departments lays out three elements of
provision for nurses in their developing role, which

suggest what the general public can and should expect from nurses (RCN 1987):

- Direct access to nursing care for whoever chooses it by offering services directly to people.

- An assessment of patient problems using existing and extended skills, providing programmes of care and treatment which offer help in maintaining health and coping with illness.

- Provision of an autonomous nursing service which encompasses responsibility for accepting and discharging and in some cases referring patients to other agents.

What then of the expectations of our clientele, the general public, who have no clearly identifiable collective voice (other than by means of franchise) to articulate their satisfaction or otherwise with the existing and developing role of nurses? There is some research evidence from patients and carers that nurses can provide alternative services which carers find acceptable (Garraway and Thompston, 1982; Parkes, 1980). In their review of community nursing research, Baker and colleagues (1987) surveyed public attitudes towards extending the nurse's role, and concluded that 'nurse practitioners would have a mixed reception from general practitioners, nurses and patients, but a considerable number of all groups would support such an innovation'.

Bevan, Cunningham and Floyd (1979), reporting on a study in which patients gave their opinion of nurses taking initiatives such as seeing the patient for first screening, said the respondents were generally favourable to the nurse in her supportive role as a caring or motherly figure and to her undertaking minor clinical procedures. They were more reluctant to accept the nurse in a decision-making role, at least without some assurance either by direct experience or by information from their doctors that any developments of this kind were appropriate.

It is interesting to note that the caring, motherly role so often given to nurses by other professionals features in this study. It is another example of a model which safely places nurses in a familiar subordinate role and neutralizes the potential for intelligent nursing. The socialisation of nurses into subordinate roles, and the public image of the nurse as doctor's helper, begin early in life. Accounts by children of their perceptions of nursing have been recorded by nurse lecturers at the Polytechnic of the South Bank (1988): the results make amusing but revealing listening as they describe nurses as helping the doctor, being kind and wearing funny hats. This is bound to produce cognitive dissonance in a general public fed on popular images but then observing nurses trying to fulfil a more independent role.

Happily, patients do report satisfaction with what nursing can and does offer. Paykel and Griffith (1983), in a matched study of nurses and doctors working with psychiatric outpatients, reported that patients found the nurses to be acceptable agents of treatment and rated them above medical staff in some categories.

Patients often consult nurses by telephone, and a number of studies have looked at what advice patients seek and what they think of the advice given. Perrin and Goodman (1978) used paediatric nurses in a first-line telephone consultation activity; they reported that 'nurses consistently outperformed doctors on all criteria used in the study'. In a similar project with nurses in primary health care Strain and Millar (1971) found that nurses involved in telephone consultation gave doctors more time (time to do what is left unclear) and importantly, they considered these nurses to be safe and effective.

The British government has recently put itself forward as a guardian and advocate of patients, but has been giving mixed messages about the role of nurses. The potential for nurse practitioners and the kind of work they might do is supported by some government reports and recommendations, but subverted by others. Some reports show a disturbing trend to marginalize nursing. While nursing has sought to capitalise upon the suggestions of the Cumberlege report, which clearly identifies a new and proactive nursing role, more significant power sharing documents are less palatable. The Griffiths report on community care (1988) virtually ignored the contribution of community nurses and health visitors, and laid all means for action on the doorstep of doctors and social workers. The Acheson report (1988) provides a medical response to debates on public health, and although envisaging a renaissance for the Medical Officer for Health, does not do justice to the wider context of public health – which includes a vital local government connection and the contribution of all health care professionals. The Government White Paper on primary health care (1987) makes some equally strange assumptions about the focus of prevention and health education: one could be forgiven for believing that good work done by community nurses and health visitors had never happened.

In summary, expectations for the development of nurse practitioners are clearly heightened on the part of the profession, have some acceptance by the general public, but appear to confuse government and, if the popular medical press is to be believed, worry our medical colleagues.

We need to prepare nursing professionally for the advent of nurse practitioner status, as we are not yet professionally equipped to handle the consequences of such a major step. This proposition should build on assumptions suggested by Stilwell (1988) as a basis for her own work as a nurse practitioner. She suggested that little action could be taken unless:

- A nurse can practise safely when patients have open access to their extended skills.

- An extended/expanded role is acceptable to patients.

- An extended/expanded role is acceptable to colleagues.

Simple steps might create collective change and evolution. I offer three ideas as a way forward, namely safe practice, articulating practice activities, and responsibility for action.

Safe practice depends on proper preparation through education and skill development. The properly prepared nurse needs a safe professional framework in which to practise what has been called 'protected autonomy'. This can only be achieved by introducing clinical supervision into the profession as a whole, to enable the development of the nurse practitioner role but also beginning at first level nurse training. My definition of clinical supervision is one in which opportunity is given to analyse and discuss casework, develop new skills, establish new principles in practice, provide peer support, and reduce practice-induced stress. Nurses protect themselves from difficult work by focusing on tasks, but a nurse practitioner will face work of greater complexity and stress. Clinical supervision allows expert development and examples can be drawn from the practice of psychotherapy and clinical psychology.

The nursing profession must also adopt a means of articulating and debating practice activities (Butterworth 1988). Nurses are seldom given opportunities to develop their skills in presenting case conferences or participating fully in multidisciplinary case reviews. This basic skill must be part of the repertoire of all nurses, enabling the nurse practitioner to build on a firm professional foundation.

Nursing in the UK has a history of collective (and therefore shielded) responsibility rather than individual responsibility for action. The rise of a litigation minded public, more defensive medicine and less than total defence of assumed vicarious liability by employers brings an added complication to the developing role of the nurse practitioner. Responsibility for action, and more importantly extended action, must become part of nursing's professional baggage.

These three small yet significant steps reach deep into the heart of nursing practice and education, but form only part of the changes required.

In conclusion, unless and until our own professional house is in order, and the right educational and ideological shifts have been made, can we go hand on heart to the public and ask for their endorsement of what nurses see as an important professional development?

In our enthusiasm to develop new directions, it is always well to heed the cautionary words of Kane (1977), who suggested that professionals stake claims in promising new territory and only later dig the theoretical mines to determine whether they have struck an appropriate task.

References

Baker, G., Bevan, J., McDonnell, L. and Wall, B. (1987), *Community Nursing : research and recent developments*, London: Croom Helm.

Bevan, J. Cunningham, D. and Floyd, C. (1979), *Doctors on the Move*, Occasional Paper No.7, London: Royal College of General Practitioners.

Butterworth, C. A. (1988), *Breaking the Boundaries : new endeavours in community nursing*, Inaugural Lecture, Dept of Nursing, University of Manchester, Manchester.

Garraway, J. and Thompson, H. (1982),'Short stay surgery in orthopaedics', *Health Trends*, 14, 73-4.

Kane, R. (1977), *Competency for Collaboration, Current Practice in Family Centred Community Nursing* (eds Reinhardt and Quinn), St Louis: Mosby.

Parkes, C. (1980), 'Terminal Care : evaluation of an advisory domiciliary service at St Christopher's Hospice', *Postgraduate Medical Journal*, 56, 685-89.

Paykel, E. and Griffith, J. (1983), *Community Psychiatric Nursing for Neurotic Patients*, London: RCN.

Perrin, E. and Goodman, H. (1978), 'Telephone management of acute paediatric illness', *New England Journal of Medicine*, 281, 771-74.

Polytechnic of the South Bank (1988), Images of Nursing, Diploma in Nursing Distance Learning (Dn301/401).

Royal College of Nursing (1988), *Boundaries of Nursing : A policy statement*, London: RCN.

Royal College of Nursing (1988), *Specialties in Nursing : A report of the working party investigating the development of specialties within the nursing profession*, London: RCN.

Royal College of Nursing (1987), *RCN Response to the Consultation on Primary Health Care Initiated by the UK Health Departments*, London: RCN.

Strain, J. and Millar, J. (1971), 'The preparation, utilization and valuation of a registered nurse trained to give telephone advice in a private paediatric office, *Paediatrics*, 47, 6 1050-55.

Stilwell, B. (1988), 'Patient attitudes to a highly developed extended role – the nurse practitioner', *Recent Advances in Nursing*, 21, 82-100.

Commentary

THEO SCHOFIELD

What do we mean by a nurse practitioner? A number of attributes have been described. They include:

- A specialist nurse with more knowledge and skill in a particular area.

- A nurse who is able to make independent assessments of patients and their problems.

- A nurse to whom patients can choose to have direct access.

- A nurse whose principal focus is on health promotion and whole person care.

- A nurse who can act autonomously of doctors and of managers within a team.

- A nurse who can make an equal professional contribution in decision making or policy creation in a team.

- A nurse who can make independent referrals to other agencies.

- A nurse who is nicer and easier to talk to than a doctor!

As a general practitioner in a large and reasonably well functioning primary health care team, I have been left wondering how many of these criteria are satisfied by our health visitors, midwives, community nurses and practice nurses. Each has special areas of skill, training and knowledge; each is directly accessible to patients and all are frequently the prime carer and decision maker for individual patients. The only key attribute that is commonly missing, however, is the training required to perform simple clinical examinations – but as has been shown by Stilwell and others, this is something that many nurses are keen and able to rectify.

The Cumberlege report says, 'Nurses are at their most effective when they and general practitioners work together in an active primary health care team... This is the best means of delivering comprehensive care to the consumer'.

I believe that the key to the development of the nurse practitioner is the development of patterns of teamwork that foster mutual respect and allow professional development and autonomy for all members.

GPs and nurses share a very similar occupational culture: they are committed to cure sometimes, to relieve often, to care always, and to prevent where possible. Both have a holistic perspective, seeing individuals and their problems in the context of their whole lives, and both recognise the importance of a patient-centred style of communication. This should make working together in an effective team easier, but we have to ask why such a major problem remains.

GPs and nurses both see themselves occupying a lowly position on the totem pole and may lack the self-confidence to collaborate readily with other groups. They have separate professional institutions, separate undergraduate and postgraduate education. Until recently there have not been the financial incentives or recognition of unmet health care needs that would create pressure for the development of the role of nurses in primary care. The pioneer nurse practitioners have also lacked powerful advocates or product champions from within general practice.

Julian Tudor Hart, a leading GP, wrote that 'the critical difference between the nature of doctoring and the nature of nursing has lain in the automony of doctors and the subordination of nurses', and 'as nurses can no longer be obedient to doctors and it is still assumed that they must be obedient to someone they are now subordinate to nursing officers, many of whom no longer have personal responsibility for patient care' (Tudor Hart 1985). It is difficult for nursing members of teams to participate fully in decision making if they are hedged about by restrictions imposed on them by managers from outside.

Professor Butterworth is absolutely right to describe the ability to articulate and describe one's ideas as a basic skill which is fundamental to taking an equal role in a professional team. As he points out, the stereotype of the caring female conflicts with that of the assertive professional. The meek only inherit the earth in the next world, not this one! I have difficulty, however, with his suggestion that clinical supervision should be developed throughout nursing. The dividing line between supportive supervision and control is narrow, and is particularly difficult for superiors in a management hierarchy to maintain. His goal of professional and expert development can be much better achieved by the development of peer review, which would also have the benefit of building collaboration and confidence within teams.

Butterworth also states that nurses may be staking claims in promising new territory and that innovators are always looking for new ideas. The current gold rush is towards prevention and health promotion. We will be on much firmer ground in attempting to build the role of the nurse practitioner as a member of the primary health care team if we concentrate first on developing services for patients with chronic diseases, children, the mentally ill and people who are elderly or dying. This is the core of the challenge that faces us, and we should be doing all that we can to avoid competition and to foster collaboration in providing care for these patients.

Reference

Tudor Hart, J. (1985), 'The world turned upside down: proposals for community based undergraduate medical education', *Journal of the Royal College of General Practitioners*, 35, 63-8.

Commentary

EVELYN MCEWEN

Age Concern was grateful to be invited to discuss patients' needs since primary care professionals spend so much time with elderly people, and the future growth in their number in the UK will increase demands on the service. My perspective is based on the people who present problems to advice workers, and as part of an interest group which attempts to influence public policies.

My impression so far is that we would do well to hurry slowly, looking carefully at the role of existing health and social care professionals and the development, potential or obsolescence of features of their work, and ensuring that there is actually a place for a new professional. One method would be to introduce pilot projects although these have tended to be a curse in the present system – used by governments as demonstration of interest for limited inputs, and taking so long to evaluate that sometimes there are no conclusions available for many years.

As a voluntary organisation Age Concern must applaud innovation and the exploration of new methods of providing primary care. That is easy. But for patients, new methods may lead to confusion. At times of crisis they need to know to whom they can turn for certain services. This lesson comes home to us vividly as a national agency: for instance, not only are the names of nursing professionals different, but the places where they can be located vary from area to area. You as experts may recognise the term nurse practitioner, you have taught me about the practice nurse as an equal member of the primary care team; but the public still sees the nurse.

A fundamental review accompanied by restructuring should surely start from the patient's needs – diagnosis of medical problems; continuing support with disability and chronic illness; an understanding of the psychological, social and economic factors in their lives; understanding and involvement of the informal carers; and increasingly, the concern of individual elderly people to promote their own health. From this perspective, what matters first is not a preoccupation with professionalisation and role definition – where do practice nurse, community nurse and health visitor end and the nurse practitioner begin? – but with the skills needed to deliver specific services.

What patients sometimes see is that the system is incomplete or has broken down; the case for the nurse practitioner may lie in default by other professionals. If this is so, review must be built on an examination of the input of all relevant workers. Even if primary health care does not become synonymous with community care, the importance of all carers working together is crucial. The problem will not be solved if nurse practitioners are put forward as the panacea, leaving others out of the picture. Where there is professional rivalry, the poor patient can be left behind – my agency has been concerned in the past that it might lead to general practitioners using fewer of their skills on the care of the elderly.

Organisations who do not see themselves as experts rely on professionals to help them determine attitudes and speak to policy makers on behalf of their interest groups. When there are obvious dissonances we stand aside, or are buffeted by whichever ear we happen to be closest to when making our decisions. We may also waste time which could be more usefully deployed holistically. Faced with the incessant demands of patients who have difficulties with their GPs, we spent two years evolving a set of guidelines with GPs, which puts upon them many of the responsibilities that Barbara Stilwell outlined in her seven points.

If the nurse practitioner is not merely filling gaps but offering a new service to patients, can we identify what that will be, or will other professional groups accept that they relinquish areas of care? We have already identified groups in the USA who may have been isolated from the traditional health system – drug addicts, AIDS victims – but who can be sustained by different structures and care workers. It would be valuable if nurse practitioners and the primary care team were viewed in relation to different client groups. Underlying the role is the question of generic as opposed to specialist client group workers. Will there be a nurse practitioner for everyone or will we be calling in future years for a geriatric nurse practitioner? In certain health and social professions the preponderance of interest ignores elder care, and less trained and skilled workers are left to provide support.

Positively nurse practitioners would increase choice and may offer new skills and services to patients. Their attitude to patients could lead to a new dimension of support for carers, where medical ethics preclude doctors fully involving carers and sometimes lead to their being ignored. Direct access to health visitors has been a boon to Age Concern in advising elderly people, and to families who despair of support, or even interest, from their GP.

An action plan for patients must concentrate on standards of care and accessibility to that care. Recent British practice has focused on the former, evolving codes of practice and guidelines, and we have neglected access. If a new profession is introduced, it would certainly have to be accompanied by far more information about the system than is currently easily available over the country.

I hear voices saying that progress achieved by such methods goes at a snail's pace. Starting from an honest look at the failures in the present system, more might be achieved for the patient this way, particularly if it is the professionals who get together and decide whether the nurse practitioner has a place and what it should be. Ultimately, the case to the patient must be made in human terms – transmogrifying Nerys Hughes from a 1930s district nurse into a late twentieth-century nurse practitioner.

7 An ideal consultation

BARBARA STILWELL

Following a study to explore the contribution a nurse practitioner can make to primary health care in a general practice setting (Stilwell, Greenfield, Drury and Hull, 1987), a further three-year study was designed to provide a functional definition of a nurse practitioner in general practice in Britain.

Eleven nurses were observed during 339 consultations in general practice, and interviews were conducted with clients, nurses and doctors, to ascertain their views on the usefulness of an expanded role for nurses in general practice. Results showed that most nurses established friendly and warm relationships with their clients. They used the consultation time for health teaching and exploration of clients' attitudes to treatment and follow-up. Clients appreciated the time they felt the nurse gave them, the friendly style of consultation and the information given. There was considerable support for the developing nursing role from medical practitioners, particularly for their contribution to facilitating health understanding and the long-term care of people with chronic problems.

Key principles

The results of this study provided the framework of an 'ideal' nursing consultation in general practice, which could be a model for the nurse practitioner role.

The complexity of care given by nurse practitioners is a characteristic feature of the role. It may result from a presentation which is, in itself, complicated. This may be a vague a complaint such as 'I don't feel well' or quite specific, such as haemoptysis. These presentations require the nurse to collect and sort information and, based on an assessment, make a decision regarding the client's future care.

Nurses with less extended roles have simpler problems to sort out, such as a dressing or an infection. In these cases the task tends to be the focus of the consultation. For a nurse practitioner, however, the whole person, who is a patient for the moment, is the focus of care. In the study this process was observed when nurses asked patients to 'tell their story' or asked about their family. It follows that a nurse practitioner must have the knowledge and skills to initiate nursing treatment.

There is a need for clarification of 'nursing' in this context. Fagin argues that primary care is nursing's major focus: 'The care of people with actual or potential health problems and manipulation of the environment to contribute to optimal health have been seen as the generic base of nursing practice for as long as nursing practice has been described' (Fagin, 1981: 23). Ellis (1982) suggests that nursing focuses on the person as affected by the illness while medicine focuses on the illness and its cure. Nursing, she argues, is concerned with achieving and maintaining a healthy state. Warner (1982) says nursing in primary care aims to help people cope with illness and increase their ability to do so.

In some of the consultations observed in the study it was possible to identify health teaching designed to help people cope with present illnesses and avoid future disease. Nurses focused on the person, not the disease, as is evident in comments from patients about their care. Nursing treatment concerned not only the presenting problem, but also had a long-term goal agreed with the client to achieve a healthier status. Ellis has said: 'Nursing has much to do with supporting, maintaining or enhancing human capacities for living or meeting life crises ... these possibilities are far beyond problem-solving' (Ellis 1982: 409).

Although problem-solving is a necessary part of nursing care, the process of care must involve more if it is to be effective for patients. Patients in the study appreciated time given to them, explanations, particularly in the management of their illnesses, and the warmth of the nurse. This nurse-patient relationship may be viewed as part of nursing care and important to good outcomes for patient. Peplau (1952) has already described the importance of the nurse-patient relationship.

Nursing intervention, as well as centring around a relationship, may also involve decisions regarding treatment. Nurses in this study commonly asked for patients' opinions about their treatments and about other procedures. Such a style of practice, accepting patients as partners in care, may result in decisions which do not accord with those made previously by doctors. The autonomy of this nursing role is reflected in the ability of the nurse practitioner to present and justify patients' views and decisions made during nursing consultations. Such practice requires adequate knowledge to carry out effective first contact assessment and certain treatments: in this study this includes skills of physical examination and occasionally of prescribing.

The outcomes of using such skill for nursing are different from those in medicine; the nurse aims to plan suitable and safe nursing interventions with the client. The focus for care is the client, not solely the disease and its cure. Assessment and treatment are therefore broader based and include a concern with non-medical aspects of disease, such as enhancing understanding, long-term care or rehabilitation, and the social and emotional effects of illness.

Nurse practitioners should have the autonomy to organise their own work, both in terms of time management and in following up the care of patients. Autonomy should not compromise teamwork: patients prefer doctors and nurses to work together (Stilwell 1987) and this study showed that doctors are accepting of nurses developing the scope of their practice.

The main functions of a nurse practitioner

From this and other research cited earlier, certain key functions are needed for an extended nursing role to prove satisfactory for clients, nurses and doctors.

1. Direct access to nursing care may be required for patients, and continuing care when necessary. In this study patients, nurses and doctors all acknowledged the importance of this service, both to provide for so-called trivial complaints and to help people with social or emotional problems.

2. The ability to carry out a comprehensive assessment of a person's physical, mental and emotional health is a necessary part of first-contact primary health care. A full examination such as this requires expertise in techniques of physical examination not normally taught to nurses inBritain. These techniques include the use of a stethoscope to auscultate the chest, use of an auroscope for ear, nose and throat examination, and skill in palpation. Familiarity with common investigative procedures and their use is a necessary component of this work.

3. Nurse practitioners are required to interpret their findings on full examination. This means the ability to discriminate between normal and abnormal findings and to understand the implication of the findings in terms of urgency of referral to others, particularly for medical or surgical treatment.

4. Most nurses in general practice now incorporate health 'teaching' in their consultations, and adequate skills to promote understanding are important for nurses in this setting. Preventive work – focusing on long-term health – seems to be an integral function of this nursing role, for nurses, patients and doctors. The nurse practitioner should be able to organise and carry out screening programmes, understand epidemiological statistics   and their relevance to practice, understand the techniques of effective education for all age groups, and know what screening is appropriate for each.

5. Consumers value the accessibility and approachability of nurses in general practice. A nurse practitioner can be a first contact for people who feel most comfortable talking to a nurse. Such consultations provide opportunities for health education as well as counselling. Nurse practitioners require social and communications skills to ensure ease of rapport.

6. A nurse practitioner needs the ability to advise, prescribe and carry out appropriate nursing treatments. These may be interventive, such as medication, or supportive, such as counselling or teaching. All respondents felt that nurse practitioners should be able to prescribe from a limited list of drugs, knowing side-effects, therapeutic effects, contra-indications and dosage of all drugs used. Further education in pharmacology will be necessary for most nurses. Patients will continue to depend on nurses for practical nursing procedures and these are already part of nurses' skills. Many nursing interventions which teach people how to cope with their illness are particularly appropriate for certain groups of patients such as the chronic sick or the elderly, and nurse practitioners

should be aware of ways in which nursing care may improve the quality of care for particular groups of patients.

Conclusion

This paper has defined a role for nurse practitioners based on the preliminary results of research which identified some key factors of nursing practice which are important for clients. Although the sample was small, previous research supports the findings.

The role of the nurse practitioner is not defined solely by transference of tasks, but by an autonomy of practice involving case management and time organisation. A nurse practitioner is concerned with the past, present and future care of all aspects of a person's health and takes responsibility for the care given, as well as its outcomes. There are legal implications for this extended role which involve changes in the law relating to prescribing. Indemnity for practice will also need close scrutiny.

References

Ellis, R. (1982), 'Conceptual issues in nursing', *Nursing Outlook*, July/August, 30, 406-10.

Fagin, C. (1981), 'Primary care as an academic discipline', In Mauksh (ed.) *Primary Care: A contemporary nursing perspective*, New York: Grune & Stratton.

Peplau, H. (1952), *Interpersonal Relations in Nursing*. New York: Pitman.

Stilwell, B., Greenfield, S., Drury, V. and Hull, F. (1987), 'A nurse practitioner in general practice: working styles and pattern of consultations', *Journal of the Royal College of General Practitioners*, 37, 154-57.

Stilwell, B. (1987), *Patients' Attitudes to the Availability of a Nurse Practitioner to General Practice*, Chichester: John Wiley.

Warner, M. (1982), *Health and Nursing: Evolving one concept by involving the other*, Nurse Paper 13, 10-17. School of Nursing, McGill University, Montreal, Canada.

Commentary

GEOFFREY RIVETT

I became interested in nurse practitioners three years ago when transferred to my present job as head of the medical division in the Department of Health concerned with primary health care. In a new field like this a variety of views co-exist; my own may change and do not, in any case, represent departmental policy.

The term 'nurse practitioner' is being used increasingly by primary health care teams. In 1989 I met a number of nurse practitioners in the USA and Raymond Kaye, a eminent figure in Kaiser Permanente in Southern California, who had been involved in the early developments. Kaiser rapidly realised that training nurses to perform broader clinical roles in physician-nurse had advantages in primary care and nurse practitioners could also work effectively in obstetrics, gynaecology paedicatrics and medicine. Others have, perhaps simplistically, said that it is at the two ends of life, with the old and the young, that nurse practitioners are most useful.

I would like to make three points on role – the issues of boundary setting, responsibilities, and protocols; education; and autonomy.

First, the role. It is easier to say what a nurse practitioner is not than what she is. She is not a physician's assistant carrying out procedures purely at the request of the doctor, nor is she a nurse specialist as I understand the term, although nurse specialists have some of the same characteristics. For example, both have an extensive knowledge of a defined specialty and evidence of relevant postbasic study. The Chief Nursing Officer (Department of Health, UK) recently suggested that a nurse practitioner was a nurse, midwife or health visitor who, in association with medical colleagues and with relevant training and experience, undertakes a wide range of health activities that best meet the needs of particular client groups or the community. This is a helpful starting point although it is arguable that we could go further; otherwise most nurses could use the title and the concept slips through our fingers.

We should be clear whether we are talking about a professional development in nursing, or a professional development in health care. Is the nurse practitioner no more than a well educated nurse, or has she a new craft? If the former, nurse practitioners are essentially a matter for the nursing profession. If the latter we all, including Parliament, need a say. Perhaps as the Americans invented the term, we ought to use it as they use it – and not hijack it to mean something quite different. My own working definition is that a nurse practitioner is a clinician who, on the basis of nurse training and experience, has been educated and has developed the skill to diagnose and prescribe care on a regular basis for particular groups of patients, within the protocols of a medical unit of which she is an integral part and to which she is accountable.

Because I am accused of a heresy known as 'adopting the medical model' I point to the definition of medicine in the Oxford Dictionary as 'the art of restoring and preserving health'. Nursing workers sometimes consider medicine to be a limited and mechanistic activity. Few doctors would recognise some nursing descriptions of doctors' activities. From the doctor's point of view, a number of nursing concepts are themselves hard to comprehend; for example, 'nursing intervention'. 'Intervention' is clear enough but what makes a 'nursing' intervention special? Then there is a stress on 'sickness' and 'health' agendas. Sir John Simon was sorting out cholera in London, clearly a 'health agenda', before Florence Nightingale was back from the Crimea: care for the public health is a traditional and vital component of medicine, a belief that Simon and Nightingale both held passionately.

There are several characteristics of the nurse practitioner but not all are mandatory. There must be an element of independent decision making at first contact, even though this takes place within a team and is guided by protocols. There may be direct access by the patient to the nurse practitioner. There is an ability to reach a diagnosis and to treat at least the simpler and common conditions. And there is a holistic ethos and a feel for continuing care.

Barbara Stilwell has shown that most nurses establish friendly and warm relationships with their clients. She has shown that nurses give people the time they need; and that is as it should be. But talk-in programmes on the radio give people time too, as do psychiatrists, psychotherapists and counsellors. So giving time is not uniquely a nursing attribute. Granted that 'consumer acceptance' is a good thing, this does not get us far. Patients like many things, not all of which are good for them.

Stilwell's paper talks about an expanded role for nurses in general practice. It refers to collecting information, assessing it and deciding about future care. Larry Weed said the same thing about the problem-oriented approach to medicine, obtaining subjective statements from the patient, an objective assessment of physical findings, an analysis and a plan for care. Both define the role of the nurse practitioner and the doctor identically. Stilwell's definition sounds very much like the Royal College of General Practitioners' definition of GPs. She is opting for parallel working of nurse practitioner and doctor and by implication sees the nurse practitioner as essentially different from other nurses, specialist or not.

The role of the nurse practitioner in primary care may concentrate, as Stilwell says, on health promotion and on the long-term care of people with continuing problems.

I suspect that continuity and empathy are essential components. Nurse practitioners make systems work better and work cheaper. There is personal warmth, and they may perform non-technical procedures better than doctors. They identify and cover the gaps left by the doctor. This is more than sweeping up boring jobs; it is the identification of crucial activities that others are missing. Nurse practitioners are not doctors manque. They are a parallel and complementary form of provision with an emphasis on continuity and completeness rather than a difference in work content.

Neither must confuse functions with responsibilities. Legislation can define responsibilities; it exists in the USA and ultimately it may be important to define the powers and responsibilities of the nurse practitioner in statute in the UK. There is generally a need for protocol in the clinical teams in which nurse practitioners work. The Cumberlege report on community nursing stressed the desirability of a clear statement of the objectives of each team member. In the patient's interests doctors and nurses should draw up protocols for care, to which all are bound and which define the overlaps and the point at which the nurse practitioner and the doctor consult each other. The midwives did this some years ago and they are probably the best UK example of a nurse practitioner.

Secondly, education. It is generally accepted that anyone caring for patients, nurse or doctor, should be trained for the job. In the USA the future nurse practitioner must have a good clinical background before entering training. It may not be right to say, as the American Nurses' Association does, that entry should be restricted to those with a degree; most British nurses who are suitable for training do not have such a qualification and should not be excluded.

Nurse practitioner training must have a strong vocational component. In the USA it combines an academic element, didactic tuition and supervised clinical experience. On the basis of a clear definition of the specialty in which the nurse practitioner is to work, education is designed to meet that goal. Training will certainly involve a deeper knowledge of psychology, social sciences, clinical pharmacology, anatomy, physiology, and the techniques of history-taking and examination than the basic nurse education system provides. Curricula design will be difficult but many doctors are keen to help. Nurse practitioners cannot rely on empathy alone or they will be lethal.

A final point on autonomy, a word by groups trying to determine their own identity – it is an illusory concept. My dictionary defines autonomy as 'the right of self-government, freedom of will'. Nurses sometimes seem to mean 'the right to take a decision without checking with anyone else'. The word is more frequently used than defined. Groups as important as health professionals should not claim the right to govern themselves without the statutory powers I have referred to.

In practice, those who claim autonomy may be unwise to do so, for there comes a time when one's knowledge and facilities do not meet the needs of the patient. GPs are obliged under their Terms of Service to refer patients to hospital services when needed; nor do doctors have unfettered autonomy in deciding treatment. If facilities are lacking they cannot be ordered. No doctor can believe that there are no constraints or that somebody else may not help the patient better. Let us hear less talk of autonomy and more of working together.

Nurse practitioners ultimately have to be seen as part of a particular hierarchy. Perhaps they should be on the medical budget and part of a clinical team and not, like a nurse specialist, on the nursing establishment; if so there are territorial issues to handle.

In conclusion, the nurse practitioner has an important role, and the next ten years will see her arrival in significant numbers, at least in primary care. What we now need is professions working together to define the role, the protocols within which the nurse practitioner operates the necessary training, and the group in which the work will be carried out. We are not here to throw mud at each other's disciplines because for every medical misdemeanour there is also a nursing one. Patient care is a team game, not to be undertaken in glorious isolation. There is no question that the nurse practitioner moves across current boundaries into the traditional territory of the medical profession. I am not in favour of job demarcation so I welcome this. I only hope that in taking on new and exciting roles nurses are not too proud to learn as they enter new fields to the benefit of patients.

Commentary

BARBARA ROBOTTOM

The title 'nurse practitioner' causes confusion. Project 2000 describes the nurse at the end of the period of preparation as a registered practitioner, and therefore by implication a practitioner of nursing. This seminar is discussing a practitioner of nursing, midwifery or health visiting, who is to be found not solely in the primary health care setting.

Barbara Stilwell has given us definitions of nursing by Fagin, Ellis and Warner. These accord with and develop the more commonly used definitions based on Henderson (1966) and indeed on the teachings of Florence Nightingale; all stress the focus of care as the client, and emphasise working with the client. This implies accepting patients as partners. If any nurse follows these ideals, her work cannot or should not be task oriented.

The focus of care on the client should be so for all health care professionals; the 'whole person' is not the prerogative of the nurse practitioner. I therefore question Stilwell's statement that we are talking about an extended role of the nurse. Surely the role is one which has been propounded for many years? However, I accept that the role has not been brought to fruition in many places and for various reasons.

What is different about the nurse practitioner as described by Stilwell? Time is constantly mentioned: the average nurse practitioner consultation is twenty-two minutes, against six minutes for a doctor. We have heard clear reasons why it can be preferable for the client to see a nurse, but we must not presume it is a cheaper option. However, there seems to be a clear case for saying it is more cost effective in the long term if the extra time is used to teach patients self care, allay fears, relay information on available resources, and so on.

So, who is the nurse practitioner? Stilwell has identified the main functions, but I have difficulty in identifying it as an extended role; what is being described is nursing as it should be. All these functions, except physical assessment and, at present, prescribing, can or should be carried out by district nurses, health visitors or community psychiatric nurses and others. They are equipped to undertake this role through their extensive post-registration programmes. Most of these courses have common elements which concentrate on assessment skills (except for a medicalised approach to physical assessment), planning, implementation and evaluation of care. This includes assessment of the health care needs of the community, the family and the individual. Health teaching, communication skills and accountability are also well covered. Following the recommendations in the government White Paper on primary health care, work is being undertaken on nurse prescribing.

If these programmes do equip nurses for this role, why have people undertaken research to show a need for the nurse practitioner? As indicated earlier a key element is time, and I would argue we require more of what have got rather than a new role. In the White Paper the government admitted that there was not one extra district nurse than ten years previously. Nurses leave their year-long courses with clear ideals of how they should function, but find they are constrained to crisis-style working; hence the potential for the development of a new worker to plug the gap.

We need not only more people, but also a loosening of the organisational structure to enable people to fulfil the roles for which they are educated and trained. All appropriately qualified community nurses should be free to undertake a more independent role, although no health care professional works totally independently – there is always a degree of interdependence, that is, partnership in care. Many interesting developments along these lines have taken place since the publication of the Cumberlege report, White Paper and Project 2000. Pre-registration nurse preparation programmes will have a focus on health promotion and health teaching, providing a different basis for post-registration courses.

Not all community nurses will wish, or be required to undertake the role described by Stilwell. Some will develop expertise in areas such as child abuse or pain control; these nurses with a specialist role will be different from but as important as the person who specialises in a nurse practitioner role.

I observed the work of a range of community nurses in the USA in 1987, and I did not see the nurse practitioner do anything that was not undertaken by other community nurses. The nurse practitioner in the USA is educated to masters degree level, but it is interesting to note that a district nurse educated at a polytechnic in England who applied to do a masters degree for nurse practitioners in the USA received exemption from the whole course, except the module on physical assessment, on the basis of having completed the district nursing course.

In summary, therefore, the role as described is essential for the consumer and should ultimately be cost effective. It is not an extended role, but an existing and progressive role for community nurses who have undertaken post-registration courses. There are staff qualified to undertake the role (with the exception of some physical assessment skills and nurse prescribing), but we need more of them and we need a different organisational structure to enable the role to be fulfilled.

Reference

Henderson, V. (1966), *The Nature of Nursing*, London: Collier MacMillan.

8 Medical perspectives

RONALD KING

All is not well with the NHS. It has grown up, understandably, in a largely autonomous manner, responding to change in demography, epidemiology, public demand and professional opinion with little in the way of overall control. To some extent this is inevitable; such a service must be responsive. At the same time it should not be at the mercy of either the providers or the recipients of health care. Easily said, but such a view is liable to produce a head-on collision between the proponents of freedom and the advocates of control. Freedom for patients to choose? For the professions to lead? Or control, and if so, by whom?

If the visions of those two health care innovators of the 1940s, William Beveridge and Aneurin Bevan, are to be fully realised, there needs to be a significant modification of attitudes. The medical profession must accept the need for change and should forswear to some extent the sanctity of clinical freedom, the nursing hierarchy welcome a more extended role, and the general public accept more readily what health services are needed, not demanded and where and how they should be provided. The necessity for such attitudinal change has been highlighted by Stocking (1985), who doubts its happening. She said, in relation to the development of nurse practitioners, 'To what extent the nursing and medical professions will allow this to happen is questionable'.

The professions are, however, becoming increasingly conditioned to the need for evaluation, for audit and for change, as evidenced by the confidential enquiries into maternal and prenatal deaths and, more recently, into perioperative mortality. What has yet to be fully acknowledged is the requirement to look at both new and traditional health service practices to determine their impact on patient outcome and their cost; in other words, cost/quality assessment. The consequence of this failure is a significant misuse of resources, the service suffering not only from financial malnutrition but also a significant degree of financial malabsorption.

It is known that bio-chemical investigations increase at an annual rate of 10 per cent with no parallel patient benefit, that pre-operative chest X-rays are frequently requested unnecessarily, and that buildings in the shape of hospital accommodation are misused by inordinate lengths of stay (Anderson *et al*, 1988). Sophisticated technologies such as CAT scanners have been introduced without preliminary evaluation, and many drugs are ineffective, not taken or even positively harmful. The King's Fund consensus conference on the treatment of patients with terminal cancer was left in no doubt on this score (Smith, 1988). But the most expensive resource lies not in investigations, buildings, machines or drugs, but in people. It is in the misuse of personnel that the NHS is most at fault. Throughout the UK tasks are performed daily which are wholly inappropriate to the professional expertise of those concerned. Such duties could be carried out as effectively by others and in many cases more effectively and certainly more economically, with skills developed for those specific purposes. The NHS has a major demarcation problem, if not a dispute, on its hands; a state of affairs more extensive in scale and wider in scope than that which plagued British industry in the late 1960s.

When the Princess Royal visited the British Postgraduate Medical Federation in 1988 she was shown a range of topics currently included in postgraduate programmes. Her Royal Highness was not impressed, her immediate comment being 'Why don't you train the nurses to do most of these tasks?' Looking at the NHS from the outside, dispassionately, as a non-expert, Her Royal

Highness pinpointed a significant problem. It applies not only to general practice. The concept itself and the issues raised, have ramifications throughout the whole of the NHS and indeed the world. Nurse practitioners are just the tip of the iceberg. The Princess raised the question of delegation. Who does what? Why? Does it need doing? And most important of all, could it be done as well or even better by someone less skilled?

Change in the NHS is notoriously difficult to achieve, reflecting Newton's third law of motion, 'Action and reaction are equal and opposite'. Opposing reactions will come from the professions and their organisations, from educational bodies, the general public and, when parochial issues are concerned, from their representatives in Parliament.

What then are the perspectives of doctors on this controversial issue – the nurse practitioner? A lifetime devoted to the NHS in general practice, as a consultant physician, in medical administration and with medical education and research provides an appropriate background for a bird's-eye view.

Opinions from general practice are predictably mixed. Many practitioners will admit to being involved in too much trivia; at the same time there is resistance to interference from outside. Some see nurse practitioners as an intrusive threat to their traditional role, whilst others consider them to be unnecessary. Many admit to a fear of change, to the practice itself or to their personal independence and status; an anti-hierarchical attitude encourages rigidity and isolation.

Some doubt the competence of nurses to take over any of the doctor role, others fear breaches of confidentiality or have misgivings about such practicalities as space and expense. Professional bodies have not been helpful with regard to responsibility or legal implications and there is a real fear that the doctor/patient relationship may be impaired. Such anxieties overlook the fact that modern health care is the result of a team effort, the proper functioning of the team as a whole being, on occasions, more important than the performance of a particular individual, even the doctor. Despite these possible objections many practitioners welcome the opportunity for change, particularly younger members of the profession.

Consultants tend to remain detached. 'It is not our business.' Like the general practitioners and the public they are averse to change, they fail to recognise nurses as equals and still cherish independence and clinical freedom. Others do see the need for increasing delegation, particularly in areas such as intensive care, where nurses have an indispensable role, and welcome a similar trend in general practice.

To the man or woman in the street (and to many professionals) the answer to Health Service problems is more money. But as Sir Brian Thwaites, former chairman of the Regional Health Authority has pointed out (1987) financial input will never keep pace with increasing demand. A real annual growth of 0.5 per cent competing with demand increasing at ten times this rate will, in ten years, result in a cumulative deficit of 50 per cent. Undoubtedly additional money is required but better use must be made of the current provision.

Manpower imbalance might appear to be of no concern to the champions of the nurse practitioner, but there is an important relationship. The excessive number of junior doctors is a response to uncontrolled patient demand with more patients attending hospital, while consultant numbers have not increased proportionately. The workload has been largely taken on by the juniors, often inappropriately. But where should patients be seen, and by whom?

There is a need to shift the load from hospital to primary care and change the pattern of work for all grades, nurse practitioners included. The old to new out-patient ratio is far too high, more day cases would lower in-patient numbers, the development of day centres could reduce out-patient work load and a proportion of consultant work (especially follow-up) could revert to general practitioners. Juniors should ideally only undertake duties appropriate for their training.

General practitioners could not meet this increased burden without delegating and modifying their own working practices, increasing the number of practice managers, practice nurses and nurse practitioners. As Project 2000 envisages, nurses themselves could delegate work to nursing aides. The nurse practitioner may be just one link in this chain of delegation and change but she/he is absolutely essential for its implementation.

Shifting the load would also have significant educational implications not only to demonstrate the need, but also to effectively equip those taking on new tasks. General practitioners would accept more continuing care of their patients, and nurse practitioners could shoulder their share of the load from the principals in their practices.

Before such developments can occur, however, there is a need for more fact-finding, health service operational research. Is the work of a senior house officer clearly defined? Is it effective and is it necessary for him/her to do it? Could another professional do it as well or better at less cost? The same questions could be asked of all staff working in health care, and the answers could form the basis for a fresh approach to the use of personnel. New structures and working patterns could be tested in trials in selected districts. The nurse practitioner concept, approached in this way, could provide a model for the promotion of delegation and teamwork, leading to a more effective use of NHS staff, greater cost-effectiveness and increased job satisfaction.

Trollope said in his autobiography (1883), 'No man can work long at any task without considering much, whether that which he daily does tends to evil or to good'. All who work in the NHS could well look at what they are daily doing and, like Trollope, decide whether their activities could be directed to better effect.

This would require an overall change in attitudes leading to a modification of referral and attendance patterns, alterations in job content and a better use of resources. Why not use the nurse practitioner as a model, and make the trial district a proving ground?

The questions to be asked are not 'What should nurses do?' but rather 'What tasks need to be done, who can do them most effectively and economically, and in what way can nurses help?'

References

Anderson, P. *et al* (1988), 'Use of hospital beds', *British Medical Journal*, 297, 910-12.

Smith, A. (1988), 'Consensus on overtreating cancer', *British Medical Journal*, 297, 438.

Stocking, B. (1985), *Initiative and Inertia: Case studies in the NHS*, London: Nuffield Provincial Hospitals Trust.

Thwaites, B. (1987), *The NHS: The end of the rainbow*, Southampton University: Institute of Health Policy Studies.

Trollope, A. (1883), *An Autobiography*, London: Blackwood.

Commentary

JOHN CHISHOLM

As one of only two practising general practitioners participating in this seminar, I feel rather like a cannibal invited to the annual meeting of the Vegan Society. Not only is there a perception that GPs might if unrestrained eat nurse practitioners for breakfast, but I also hear some nurses express the view that nurses and doctors have completely different diets, with doctors thriving on illness and dealing with patients according to a medical model, while only nurses can enjoy the true nourishment of health promotion and health education and practice in a holistic manner.

Ronald King suggests that a major obstacle to change in the NHS is the entrenched professional self-interest of doctors, who he suggests have a Newtonian 'equal and opposite reaction' to each and every innovative proposal for service improvement. Yet the views that doctors are wedded to a National Illness Service, are not interested in prevention and are irrationally conservative are fallacious generalisations.

There is uncertainty about the very meaning of the term 'nurse practitioner'. Perceptions of what a nurse practitioner is vary within the UK, but they vary even more widely between other countries, some of which have more experience of nurse practitioner care than we do. We hope our present discussions will help to clarify the concept, but it is already quite plain that the acceptance of a new nursing role will depend on the particular health care system in which it might be exercised.

The practice organisation subcommittee (which I chair) of the General Medical Services Committee of the British Medical Association has within its remit the roles of employed and attached staff in general practice, while the

General Medical Services Committee is the only body that represents all NHS general practitioners. Dr King, while praising the openness to change of some GPs, painted many doctors and their professional organisations as resistant to new ideas. There is evidence, though, that suggests the contrary.

First, the GMSC in its evidence to the Cumberlege review of community nursing in England recognised that each member of the primary health care team had a proactive role, and that reactive situations where the demand for care had been initiated by the patient still afforded opportunities for prevention and patient education (BMA, 1986a). We said patients should be able to consult a community nurse directly whenever they wished, rather than through their GP, while pointing to the need to share information within and for referral within the team when another member's care was more appropriate.

Second, in response to the government's consultation document *Primary Health Care – An Agenda for Discussion* (BMA, 1986b) and to the Cumberlege report, we welcomed an extended role for nurses, so as to increase their responsibility and professional satisfaction, with the development of new skills leading to an increased service to the community and greater involvement in health education and preventive care. We noted, however, that

in many respects the duties and responsibilities of the nurse practitioner as described in the Cumberlege report resemble those of the practice nurse. But the term 'nurse practitioner' remains ill-defined and nursing organisations do not appear to have reached agreement among themselves on a common usage. We would welcome further clarification.

Meanwhile the General Medical Services Committee has been having positive discussions with the Royal College of Nursing about nurse prescribing, producing a joint statement in December 1987 (BMA, 1988) and giving evidence to the government's advisory committee on nurse prescribing that demonstrated our common cause with the RCN. We acknowledge that nurses working in the community experience difficulties in obtaining appropriate supplies of medicines, dressings and appliances and that decisions about appropriate treatment are in practice not always made by a patient's GP. We have therefore made proposals including a national nursing formulary, assessment of competence to prescribe, and protocols for care, which should ensure that patients enjoy better and more timely care. We still believe that 'patients will continue to expect that their doctor will have overall responsibility for any medical treatment they receive. Any extension to the present circumstances in which nurses have the right to prescribe will need to take account both of these expectations and the doctor's responsibility for the patients in his care.' Nonetheless, we believe that change is essential. Change includes acceptance of a change in roles, and we are keen to see proper arrangements, including where necessary legislative arrangements, to accommodate it.

The prescribing issue is a good example of the acceptance by the representatives of general practice of changing roles in the primary health care team, with an extension of the nurse's role. But it is not the only such example – for instance, together with the Health Visitors' Association we have been examining the health of homeless families, and among a large number of recommendations in our forthcoming report we acknowledge that the health visitor has the crucial role in facilitating access to primary care for these families.

Whether we are talking about further extensions of the work of the practice nurse, including open access by patients, greater autonomy and independent professional responsibility within team protocols – or an entirely new entity, two points are clear. First, there is a need for proper training. We have pointed out the major implications for the training of nurses if significant extensions of nurse prescribing are made. Any professional has a duty to obtain appropriate training and to acquire knowledge, skills and the necessary competence before undertaking any task or new role.

Second, there is a need for for proper remuneration of nurses undertaking an extended role. Practice nurses vary widely in their experience, the tasks they undertake and the autonomy they accept. Through the ancillary staff scheme, NHS GPs have had the resources to pay whatever is necessary to attract staff of the right calibre in the context of the local job market. Seventy per cent of those salaries is reimbursed to them directly, while the 30 per cent that GPs bear individually acts as a cost constraint to ensure that they are not profligate. While the pay scales suggested by the review body on nurses' pay can serve as useful guidelines, GPs as independent contractors have the scope and the right to set appropriate salaries for their practice nurses. It is particularly unfortunate and unnecessary that some family practitioner committees are now seeking to limit GPs' reimbursements under the ancillary staff scheme, in effect limiting what GPs can pay nurses undertaking extended roles. This development is one factor that may militate against the spread of nurse practitioners in the UK, for they might not receive the remuneration they deserve.

Finally, I welcome Dr King's suggestion that there is a need to examine the appropriateness of the current division of labour in the NHS. While I do not share Trollope's confidence that all men consider the consequences for good or evil of their daily tasks, it is right that all of us should do so. The examples of the evaluation of care that Dr King gives are audit by peer review, which I believe is the proper way forward. The need for external audit and control should only be considered when peer review has demonstrably failed. The medical and nursing professions, in willingly accepting that obligation to look at their own activities, will be greatly aided by the increasing information now available about the process of care.

References

British Medical Association (1986a), 'General Medical Services Committee: Evidence to the Cumberlege review team on community nursing in England', Appendix X, 48-51, *Annual Report*, London: BMA.

British Medical Association (1986b), *General Medical Services Committee Report to Special Conference of Representatives of Local Medical Committees*, London: BMA.

British Medical Association (1988), *General Medical Services Committee Annual Report*, London: BMA.

9   Lessons for future policy

NICHOLAS BOSANQUET

This paper reviews the development of the nurse practitioner in the UK so as to draw out lessons for policy in the future. It finds that the past record has been one in which the local response has been encouraging, but that the concept has been difficult to fit to traditional views of the roles of general practitioners and of community nurses. The concluding section looks at policy options for the fuure and suggests that the most helpful types of change may well be in process and training which would give the greatest freedom to local initiative, rather than seeking to resolve national problems of definition and relative role. The future of the nurse practitioner can only be decided through local experiment and development: the policy issue at present is how to give the most opportunity for such development rather than how to pre-empt or control answers which can only emerge from local experience.

The idea of the nurse practitioner was originally American; this has perhaps contributed to a certain resistances to the idea. Even in the USA, the concept went through various changes. The original University of Colorado project aimed to expand the nurse's role in providing better and more widely available health care for children (*American Journal of Public Health*, 1978). As the role developed it became more concerned with primary health care. It was always clearly defined as a nursing role separate from that of the physician or the new grade of physician's assistant, but some of the stimulus for the development of the role came from the shortage of physicians. Thus the nurse practitioner came to be seen as an American import which could be explained in terms of the peculiar culture of the USA and its problems of securing adequate cover by physicians in poorer areas.

The nurse practitioner was stereotyped as a cut-price doctor, and it has proved difficult to shake off this image. The nurse practitioner role also developed in Canada. The progress of the role there shows that it can gain support for reasons other than a physician shortage (Jones, 1984). The term 'nurse practitioner' was defined in the 1972 Boudreau Report, after demands for expanded training of nurses had come from services working with Canadian Indians and residents in the Northern territories. The report of the committee on nurse practitioners defined it as a 'nurse in an expanded role oriented to the provision of primary health care as a member of a team of health professionals relating to families on a long-term basis' (Jones, 1984). In response to this report, short courses of four to six weeks were started for qualified nurses in health sciences divisions of six Canadian universities. There was professional pressure to include the new role in basic nursing education, and by the 1980s the short courses had been discontinued and baccalaureate programmes had been extended.

By 1984 Phyllis Jones, Dean of the School of Nursing, University of Toronto, said, 'Canada relies on the graduates of its 25 University baccalaureate programmes for its supply of nurse practitioners and tends to employ nurses in roles that complement rather than supplement physician functions'. The results of the first clinical trial of nurse practitioners showed that there was real collaboration. 'While the physicians focused on diagnosis and disease, the nurse's primary attention was directed towards patients' problems and the development of the interpersonal relations and social support structures necessary to improve adherence and a sense of well-being.' The continuing course at McMaster University particularly stresses teamwork between doctors and nurse practitioners who take the course together (Stilwell, 1985).

The main local interest in Britain has been in inner city general practices. Stilwell worked in such a practice in

Birmingham, and has published an analysis of her work (Stilwell *et al*, 1987). To work as independently as possible, she received further training in physical examination techniques,the detection of abnormalities, and the management of common and acute conditions in general practice. She had her own consulting room and did not wear a uniform. Patients were offered a 20-minute consultation and were free to decide for themselves whether to see the nurse practitioner or one of the doctors. Details of consultations with 858 patients were recorded during March to August 1983. The majority (72 per cent) of the nurse practitioner's patients were women; 60 per cent of problems were classified under the 'supplementary' diagnostic category – of these half were categorised as preventive medicine, a quarter concerned advice, health instruction and education, and a fifth were for 'social, marital family problems and maladjustments'.

A total of 167 patients (19.5 per cent) were referred to other workers, of whom 103 were to the GP, 25 directly to a consultant and 25 to the social services. In 127 (14.8 per cent) of the consultations the patient received a prescription signed by the GP.

The nurse practitioner played an autonomous role concerned with advice and prevention.

Although the nurse practitioner dealt with the patients' presenting problems, she was also concerned with long-term preventive strategies, such as measuring blood pressure or carrying out cervical smears, when appropriate. Patients responded readily to prompting about life-style changes and they raised many concerns of their own.

There was also an experiment with a nurse practitioner in the East End of London, where Barbara Burke-Masters gave a service to homeless people when local GPs were not willing to do so (Sharon, 1984). 'Over 2,700 patients see Sister Burke-Masters every year: many of them are extremely disturbed and occasionally violent. They are the patients that ordinary GPs and ordinary patients would rather not have in the surgery.' This experiment seems to follow the American model of a nurse practitioner acting as a physician substitute.

There has been an experiment with a nurse practitioner role in the rheumatology out-patient clinic at Leeds General Infirmary, where three nursing sisters worked in parallel with their medical colleagues to provide nursing care as a routine part of treatment (Hill, 1984). Priority was given to teaching patients about the disease and its treatment. Patients felt they received more personal and individual attention: 'I am treated as a person rather than as a number and a disease.' Others mentioned education, advice and continuity of care from the same person at each clinic visit as advantages. There has also been a successful experiment in the accident and emergency department in Oldchurch Hospital, Romford (Tattam, 1987). With the agreement of the unit's medical staff, a nurse practitioner screens every patient coming into the department to determine if they need to see a doctor. The result has been a fall in the numbers treated by doctors and a fall in waiting times, with the numbers waiting for over two hours cut from more than half to less than 4 per cent. These were certainly successes, but the role seems to have been very different from that envisaged in the Birmingham project.

These successful experiments have taken place since the early 1980s. In fact two of them finished five years ago, in 1983; further progress has been slow.

The concept found general endorsement in the Cumberlege report, which concluded that the nurse practitioner's key tasks would be to interview patients and diagnose and treat specific diseases in accordance with the agreed medical protocols; refer to the general practitioner p a t i e n t s who have medical problems which lie outside the written protocols; be available for all patients who wish to consult the nurse practitioner; give counselling and nursing advice to patients consulting her direct or referred to her by a general practitioner; conduct screening programmes among specific age or client-groups; maintain patient-care programmes, particularly to the chronic sick; refer patients for further care to the neighbourhood nursing service.

The report recommended that the principle should be adopted of introducing the nurse practitioner into primary care. However, controversy continued into the possible role of nurse practitioners in prescribing. Research has been carried out into the current role of practice nurses and the possible future role of nurse practitioners and it was hoped that a pilot course would begin by the end of 1988 (*Nursing Standard*, 1987). Thus there would be unlikely to be more than 100 nurse practitioners by 1995.

Future policy needs to take account of likely trends in both community nursing and general practice. Community nurses are likely to face a substantial increase in workload which will have to be met despite little increase in manpower. The total number of qualified nurses may well have fallen by the mid-1990s, while demands for qualified nursing time will have become more intense and varied (Bosanquet and Gerard, 1985). There would seem to be little room for the development of a sizeable (1,000+) nurse practitioner group as a net addition to total manpower. The future of the nurse practitioner grade in community nursing appears to depend on the reorientation of some of the time of nurses in existing grades; the investment in retraining would have to be justified in terms of the additional benefits to patients.

Practice nurses play a variety of roles. Total numbers have not been increasing very much and currently stand at about 5,000. General practice is becoming divided between innovators and traditionalists: innovating practices are often larger, employ practice nurses, invest in premises through the Cost Rent Scheme and take part in the vocational training scheme. They employ practice managers, own computers and have an interest in developing new preventive services as well as the management capacity to do so (Bosanquet and Leese, 1989). In these practices the role of the practice nurse is likely to expand to take on some of the role of the nurse practitioner, as interest in preventive care and in positive health increases. It is in such practices within inner cities that successful experiments have taken place.

The greatest local interest seems to be in replacing some 'practice nurses' with nurse practitioners. But their introduction into neighbourhood nursing teams would cut across the established role of general practice and lead to further friction locally and nationally. There are a number of reasons for thinking that more progress would be made within general practice. The practice nurse role is likely to expand anyway. In this context the issues and professional roles can most easily be sorted out on a day-to-day basis. The change would not lead to any net addition to manpower. There could be local incentives to encourage taking on nurse practitioners in inner city and older industrial areas.

What kind of initiatives would most encourage local experiments? There could be some national finance for a joint course between family doctors and nurse practitioners on McMaster lines. A national programme could be established for retraining practice nurses who wished to do so. A number of practices in various parts of the country – perhaps 25 – could take part in a pilot scheme for employment of nurse practitioners. Under this proposal nurse practitioners would continue to be employed by practices and there would be reimbursement of 70 per cent of their salaries, but a code of practice should be agreed on appropriate salary rates. On this highly contentious issue of employment status it would be better to retain the status quo while leaving time and successful local joint working to bring about solutions more acceptable to all the professions. In some areas there could also be experiments by health authorities in direct employment. The concept has many merits, not least in its potential for improving services for women patients: but unless there is a clear plan for allowing local initiatives to develop, there is likely to be little progress before 1995.

This paper has set out one possible route for policy. The suggestions are made as an agenda for discussion. The need above all is for a consensus which can allow local interest and local initiative to develop.

References

American Journal of Public Health (1978), 'The nurse practitioner movement – where does it go from here?' 68,11, 1074-75, November.

Bosanquet, N. and Gerard, K. (1985), *Nursing Manpower: Recent trends and policy options*, CHE Discussion Paper No.9.

Bosanquet, N. and Leese, B. (1989), *Family doctors and economic incentives*, Dartmount: Gower.   .

Hill, J. (1984), 'Patient evaluation of a rheumatology nursing clinic', *Nursing Times*, July 2, 82, 27, 42-3.

Jones, P. (1984), 'Nurse practitioners – the Canadian experience', *Nursing Times*, Sept 19, 335-41.

Nursing Standard (1987), 'Major study in role of nurse practitioner', 489, 3, 26, March.

Sharon, H. (1984), 'Nurse practitioners with a mission', *Primary Health Care* Sept 2, 9, 14-15.

Stilwell, B. (1985), 'Lifestyle equals health', *Nursing Mirror*, 160, 17, April 24, 24-6.

Stilwell, B., Greenfield, S., Drury, M. and Hull, F. (1987), 'A nurse practitioner in general practice: working style and pattern of consultations', *Journal of the Royal College of General Practitioners*, 37, 297, 154-57.

Tattam, A. (1987), 'A practical service', *Nursing Standard*, 2, 11, 32.

Commentary

ELAINE FULLARD

Professor Bosanquet reviewed the history and development of the nurse practitioner role and gives several practical examples of local experiments which could test the role more widely in the UK. In my role as a facilitator for prevention in primary care, the key issues raised in this paper are as follows:

- The need for further research on the role, to check the wider transferability of the model.

- Will the rapidly extending role of the practice nurse and the potential for an increase in their numbers under the reimbursement scheme meet the need which the nurse practitioner would otherwise have filled?

- Sources of funding.

First, to tackle the need for further research, there is a need for a controlled trial of a small group of nurse practitioners compared with a small group of practice nurses to look at the outcomes in terms of caring and cost effectiveness. This experiment could be tested in both rural and inner city districts. To my knowledge there have not been any controls in the nurse practitioner studies to date. I realise the difficulty of measuring outcome in patient satisfaction, but it is a vital next step in the light of the extending role of the practice nurse. In the current reimbursement scheme for general practice ancillary staff, there is still the potential for employment of almost as many practice nurses as are in post at present (the national average for uptake of the FPC reimbursement scheme in general practice is 1.1 full-time ancillary staff per GP instead of the potential 2.0). The training opportunities for nurses are expanding, particularly in preventive medicine, and the English National Boards for Nursing, Midwifery and Health Visiting are approving more and more courses. There are currently twenty-two, with several more planned. Practice nurses who take on extended duties, such as responsibility for patient consultation about minor ailments, are eligible, with their employer's agreement, to be considered for a higher clinical nursing scale.

My suggestion is for an extension to the existing training and more formal recognition of a role somewhere between the traditional practice nurse and the nurse practitioner. Salary scales would reflect the differences in these roles. The University of Exeter is piloting a course for practice nurse trainers and this specialised training could provide practice nurses with extra skills and knowledge.

The third issue that Bosanquet raises is that of funding. It is essential to demonstrate the cost-effectiveness of the nurse practitioner role in the light of the expanding role of both practice nurses and general practitioners. The change in practice activities that a primary care facilitator can effect by acting as a mentor and catalyst to primary health care teams in his/her health district has been demonstrated (Fullard, Fowler and Muir Gray, 1987). The power of personal contact to influence GP behaviour has been explored (Horder, Bosanquet and Stocking, 1986) and facilitators have adopted this method of visiting practice teams (Astrop, 1988). One of the hurdles of the nurse practitioner role is its transferability: given the restricted budgets of health authorities, a compromise for meeting patients' needs could be to experiment by employing a practice nurse mentor to demonstrate whether it is possible to improve patient care within the existing structure.

In conclusion, I should like to reinforce Bosanquet's suggestion for more local experimentation in the nurse practitioner role: first to test the transferability of the model and to test its effectiveness in comparison to the extending practice nurse role; second, to look at possibilities of increasing the training provision for practice nurses in this nurse practitioner role; third, to look at the possibility of formal recognition by the National Boards – to achieve financial and professional recognition of this increase in responsibility.

References

Astrop, P. (1988), 'What the facilitator can do for the practice nurse', *Practice Nurse* 1, 13-17.

Fullard, E., Fowler, G. and Muir Gray, J. (1987), 'Promoting prevention in primary care: controlled trial of low technology, low cost approach', *British Medical Journal*, 294, 1080-82.

Horder, J., Bosanquet, N. and Stocking, B. (1986), 'Ways of influencing the behaviour of general practitioners', *Journal of the Royal College of General Practitioners*, 36, 517-21.

Commentary

SHIRLEY GOODWIN

My first response to Professor Bosanquet's paper is to refer to the Canadian definition of the nurse practitioner quoted in his review of the North American experience: 'A nurse in an expanded role orientated to the provision of primary health care as a member of a team of health professionals relating to families on a long term basis.'

This definition corresponds almost exactly with the UK experience of health visiting, district nursing and other existing community nursing roles. It is interesting to note that the subsequent expansion in baccalaureate programmes in Canada allowed these graduates to fulfil the role of nurse practitioners.

It is possible to draw a parallel between the integrated and degree courses in nursing in the UK over the last thirty years which, particularly in the early years, sought to provide nurses educated to degree level and qualifying as registered nurses, qualified district nurses and health visitors. With the development of shared learning in post-registration courses for nurses working in primary health care, particularly where these courses are situated in higher education institutions where links can be made with other health care disciplines, we can perhaps anticipate a similar process as was seen in Canada for the provision of nurse practitioners in the UK.

My second observation relates to Bosanquet's realistic prediction of manpower shortages in nursing generally contributing to substantial increases in workload for community nurses, an issue about which many of us have been concerned for some time. The option he suggests, which is to reorientate the practice of existing community nurses, is both obvious and necessary. Health visiting is at present attempting to do just that, so that the role and practice of health visitors can be more relevant and effective in the future.

One aspect of this reorientation is to relate the priorities of local health visiting services to the systematically identified health needs of the populations concerned, on the basis of the community health assessment or local health profile.

Which brings me to my third point: if it emerges that the local situation indicates the need for a nurse, for example, to take an outreach service to people finding it difficult to gain access to services provided along traditional lines, then a nurse with one of the existing community nursing qualifications – perhaps extended with additional appropriate clinical or specialist skills – can be identified to service this client group. One such model was successfully developed in the late 1970s by Brenda Lawrie, a health visitor jointly employed by two East London health authorities as a health worker for travellers. Her extended role included the administration of immunisations and the provision of family planning services (Lawrie, 1983).

I therefore agree with Bosanquet that the most helpful type of changes may be in process and training, which would give the greatest freedom to local initiatives rather than in seeking to resolve national problems of definition and relative role.

I am reminded of a remark once made by Marie-Francoise Colliere, WHO consultant on primary health care, who observed that there is often a wholly inappropriate and unnecessary preoccupation with role. 'You don't ask a baker what his role is – you ask him about the kind of bread he makes!' It is the product that matters, not a somewhat introverted concern with relative role. And the product must be fitted to customer demand.

In this context, it is vital that the future development of post-registration courses for nurses working in the community – or elsewhere for that matter – ensures optimum flexibility in the choice of modules both within courses and available on an add-on basis, so that subsequent working as a nurse practitioner is only one of a range of possible options.

The one aspect of Bosanquet's paper with which I would take issue is his view that, with the current expansion in the practice nurse role, progress to achieve the introduction of nurse practitioners is likely to be more successful within general practice. I agree this will certainly be the case if we restrict our concept of the nurse practitioner to one seen as an adjunct to primary medical care. Experiments so far undertaken in the UK illustrate how well a nurse with the skills of counselling and health promotion (often brought from health visiting) can creatively complement general medical practice, and provide a service which is safe, effective and highly acceptable to users, as well as more cost-effective.

I would also argue, however, by returning to the point about the importance of local needs informing service planning, that there are other possible models for the nurse practitioner in community nursing. These could, for example, utilise a combination of outreach health promotion and preventive activities, as well as open access health consultancy, the latter being provided on the patch in community centres and street markets as well as in existing health service premises.

The question is whether we would wish to describe these more open-ended kinds of practice in terms of a new nurse practitioner role, or simply acknowledge that they are already happening in health visiting and district nursing in some areas. If the adoption of the job title 'nurse practitioner' represents a much needed and well-deserved improvement in status for some, such as practice nurses, then why not use it? But let us not deceive ourselves that a new job title can by itself provide knowledge and skills that may already be available within the ranks of existing community nurses qualified in one or other of the primary health care nursing disciplines, and where these nurses are ready to innovate and extend their practice in ways that are aimed at meeting more effectively the health needs of local populations.

Reference

Lawrie, B. (1983), 'Travelling families in East London – adapting health visiting methods to a minority group', *Health Visitor*, 56, 26-8.

Part III

Developing Primary Health Care Nursing

10 Bringing about change

BARBARA STOCKING

The innovator makes enemies of all those who prospered under the old order, and only lukewarm support is forthcoming from those who would prosper under the new.... partly because men are generally incredulous, never really trusting new things unless they have tested them by experience.

(Machiavelli, *The Prince*)

It is worth taking a sideways look at nurse practitioners and the developing role of the primary health care nurse. Instead of assessing these roles and their contribution to health services, it is possible to look at them as examples of innovation and change. There is a considerable literature (Rogers, 1980; Stocking, 1985) on the diffusion of innovations, why some are taken up when others are not, and the way innovations spread through social systems. There is also a body of literature and experience concerned with the management of change. Here I would like to look at the developing roles of primary care nurses in those contexts.

First it is important to get at the essentials or core developments in these changing roles. Those I take to include:

- Nurses having first contact with patients and making assessments, not only of their nursing needs but also their need to see other professionals. Perhaps direct referral to other professionals (physiotherapists, social workers, etc.) or access to beds.

- Prescribing, at least to a limited extent.

- Development of preventive role.

- Developed counselling role.

Not all these facets will necessarily be included in any particular experiment/development, but overall they seem to sum up the key features. The next step is to consider them in terms of innovation characteristics.

Innovation characteristics

Rogers (1980) has summarised five key characteristics that influence individuals to accept or reject innovation. Each person who has any part in the innovation will consider these characteristics for themselves – and the answer will vary for different people. What may seem to me to be perfectly compatible with my philosophy and beliefs may be quite different for another actor in the process.

Table 1   Innovation attributes

---

1. **Relative advantage:** degree to which an innovation is perceived as better than the idea it supersedes (as perceived by each sector in the adoption process).

2. **Compatibility:** with existing values, past experience and needs of potential adopters.

3. **Complexity:** perception of use or difficulty in understanding and using the innovation.

4. **Trialability:** can innovation be tried out on a limited basis?

5. **Observability:** are the results of an innovation visible to others?

Relative advantage

The advantages and disadvantages need to be assessed for a range of people, including at minimum patients, the nurses in these developing roles, their nurse colleagues, GPs, and other members of the primary care team. Of course the responses will not be uniform across these groups since individuals vary in their willingness to change: from being venturesome and perhaps a bit maverick, through careful and deliberate, to the traditional laggards who may never take up particular changes. Nevertheless, some generalisations can be made, though they would have to be checked out with the individuals concerned in any particular location.

Patients: the evidence seems to suggest that patients are very accepting of nurse practitioners and related roles. They do not seem to mind not seeing a doctor as first contact, and they value the time that nurses can give them and the information and counselling they receive.

Nurses in the new roles: the perceptions here seem to be more varied. For some nurses the developments are perceived as a great opportunity to give a better service to patients and to provide much greater job satisfaction, with room for personal development. Others, for example some practice nurses, may be less enthusiastic; they took their jobs because they did not want a high level of responsibility and are satisfied in their role of providing a support service in a practice.

Other nurses: advantages or otherwise are more difficult to assess here but are probably as varied as those of the nurses directly involved. A key group to consider is health visitors. The focus on prevention suggests a reintegration of the health visitor and district nursing roles (which may be an advantage to patients who have often not understood the divisions and not understood why they were visited by so many different people). Health visitors may welcome this as broadening and making more sense of the nursing roles, or may fear that their own areas of expertise will become devalued. More generally, local colleagues might be expected to look at anyone setting themselves up as a nurse practitioner with some suspicion – 'what are they doing that I am not, why all the fuss?'.

GPs: the doctors are clearly a key group in determining whether the roles will be accepted because of their power in the primary care setting. Their reactions seem to have varied from the small group who are highly supportive (on the basis of giving a better service to patients and relieving the doctor of considerable work), to those who prefer the nurse to operate more traditionally in support of the doctor, and are very sceptical if not hostile to more developed roles.

Compatibility

It is not necessary to go through each of the affected groups to check how compatible the primary care nurse roles are with their own philosophies, values and routines. Much of that can be deduced already from the analysis above. The nurse practitioner type developments, however, are not simply 'add-ons' in health care which conform to existing value systems; they challenge them quite fundamentally. Perhaps the key issue concerns nurses' assessments and nurses seeing patients as first contacts. This issue has been sidestepped by suggesting that the assessments concern nursing care: however, if nurses see a patient as the first contact, at home or in the surgery, they are clearly making a more general assessment in advising the patient whether to see a doctor or other health professional. Since diagnosis is at the heart of medical practice, it is to be expected that doctors would find this the most difficult aspect to accept. At local level and more especially at national policy level, the issue seems to make both doctors and nurses nervous, yet it does need to be thought through if individual practitioners are not to find themselves in very uncomfortable positions.

Prescribing is another aspect which the medical profession has long held to itself. There is considerable resistance to nurse prescribing, even for items for which it makes practical sense. Yet at least prescribing can be negotiated to result in a specific limited list which is known to all, unlike the complexities of the diagnosis/assessment issue.

Complexity

Developing primary care nurses would not seem to be a particularly complex health care innovation in that nurses already exist in primary care and people are busy developing their own roles in their individual circumstances. Some of the understanding necessary for the full nurse practitioner role is not easy, however. There are plenty of opportunities for confusion about what the nurse will and will not do, patients she or he will or will not see. The complexity of the innovation can be overcome, but it does need some mental effort and a willingness to negotiate and compromise with colleagues.

Trialability, observability and adaptability

Some of the ideas in developing the primary care nurse can be tried out without too much commitment. However, a major change is likely to require a sort of 'paradigm shift'. Nurses in a practice can try extending roles but eventually this will require major changes in training and probably negotiation at national level of the role, status, and pay and conditions for the new practitioners. However, for those wishing to push this forward, the fact that there can be such a groundswell of local developments is helpful. It is rare that an innovation can be imposed from the top. An innovation is much more likely to be widely accepted if many people on the ground are already halfway there.

The nurse practitioner moves are at least practically observable from overseas and from experiments in this country. The drawback is that they take place in primary care, which exists more in isolated nodules than as a linked, networked system. There are, though, ways to pass messages around the system and even to make visits to other practices/health centres. These mechanisms will have to be well used for nurse practitioners and related developments to become observable.

Finally, I have included adaptability since in my own study (Stocking, 1985) a key feature in whether an idea was accepted locally concerned whether it could be adapted to fit particular circumstances. This is an interesting feature in this particular context. So far a lot of local variation has been possible but sooner or later for legal reasons, if for no other, it will be necessary to impose more order and uniformity. The innovators need to be careful in ensuring that room for local flexibility can be built in.

Strategies for change

Analysis of the innovation, or in this case a range of innovatory practice, is a good starting point to assess whether it is likely to spread rapidly without much help or whether considerable effort is needed. The superficial analysis suggests that although there are likely to be blocks and resistance, primary care nursing developments have a lot going for them. So how does one go about bringing about change?

There is a good deal of work to be done at national level. The climate of opinion must be right and the issue must be on the policy agenda. The innovators need to use other developments which may foster primary care nursing. The White Paper on primary health care is an obvious example, but assessing and promoting primary health care nursing in the context of other possibilities such as health maintenance organisations or primary care authorities is worth some thought. Just as I have done in general above, analysis is needed of the key actors at national level. Who is likely to be for, who against? Who can be convinced, who ignored? Where there are particular resistances other carrots may need to be offered – can primary care nursing be seen as part of a package in which the resistant groups get their ideas on other matters supported?

Assuming all the right things are being done nationally, the message about primary care nursing has to be disseminated throughout the system. To some extent this has been done for the general concepts and has probably already generated a climate of opinion in which the ideas are familiar. There is a problem in that the developments promoted are very diffuse; although some variation can ultimately be sustained, several themes and different models of primary care nursing cannot. It does now seem to have reached the point where some clarity and agreement about the developments is needed if the field is not going to ignore the innovation out of confusion.

Also needed for innovations to diffuse are a number of examples of how it works in practice. There have already been such examples but they are very varied, ranging from facilitators and practice nurses undertaking and auditing preventive work through to the full nurse practitioner/counsellor model. For the spread of some developments, especially the full nurse practitioner model, there is a need to sort out the legal and training issues, which will require negotiation among the professions.

For broad acceptance of new models a lot of work is required in making sure people in the system really understand what an innovation means, what its problems are and how it works in practice. This may mean the innovators spending time 'showing' the innovation to

Figure 1   Diffusion of innovation

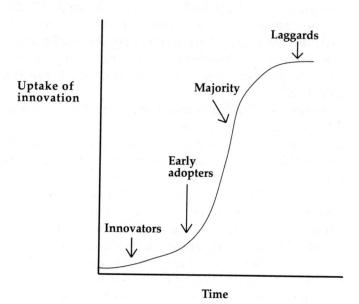

Innovators: venturesome
Early adopters: respected
Majority: deliberate ⟶ sceptical
Laggards: traditional

other people – much public speaking, roadshows, visiting, etc. This is far more difficult in primary care than in the hospital system, though drug representatives manage to get everywhere so it cannot be impossible. But if the prospect of getting to every single practice sounds daunting, other knowledge about the diffusion of innovation is more reassuring.

Somehow the ideas must get through the system. Ideas spread on networks, different people take up ideas at different stages in the diffusion process and the early adopters influence the later ones. Figure 1 shows the diffusion curve of the uptake of innovations and the characteristics of people at different stages. Once the opinion leaders in a speciality or profession have accepted the innovation, it is likely to spread throughout the system. This means it may be necessary not to reach everyone directly, but to focus attention on these opinion leaders and potential early adopters.

Evidence from both doctors and farmers suggests that opinion leaders are more cosmopolitan. They tend to go to more out of town meetings, they pick up ideas from journals and so on. They return to their own patch and it is they who convince other local adopters. The later adopters are not convinced by journal articles alone, but will wish to see what their local peers are doing, and are more convinced by word of mouth knowledge. If they are receiving the same message from many different sources – journals, local discussions, and personal contact with those who have already adopted the idea – then it gradually becomes acceptable.

Conclusion

Some innovations seem to take off by themselves, but the developments in primary care nursing are unlikely to do so. They will require considerable effort. Some understanding of the change process can help to clarify where to put the effort, which people to target, where resistance must be overcome and where it can be ignored.

The innovation itself has many ramifications and work will be needed on all fronts if it is to move forward successfully. The structural base needs to be sorted out – including the legal issues and agreement about the role and conditions of service. The financial implications need to be thought through and negotiated, and perhaps most importantly in this area, a training strategy needs to be developed. It is only then that the more direct change strategy will work successfully.

References

Rogers, E. (1980), *The Diffusion of Innovations* (third edition), New York: Free Press.

Stocking, B. (1985), *Initiative and Inertia*, London: Nuffield Provincial Hospitals.

11 The role of the regulatory body

COLIN RALPH

My approach is briefly to discuss first the semantic problems we face and the current regulatory position, second to consider the immediate challenge to the professions, and third to propose a strategy for how this development could be approached in the future. I hope to present you with a broad framework in which this development and concept should be considered.

In all that I say references to 'nurse' or 'nursing' may apply equally to 'midwife' and 'midwifery' and 'health visitor' and 'health visiting' in the UK. The UK regulatory position is a highly privileged and developed one compared with nursing in some other countries and this should not be underestimated.

Margretta Styles, author of an international report on the regulation of nursing, wrote in 1986:

As the complexities of health care and the social environment increase, nursing is in the process of creating its own destiny upon these new frontiers. In many places nursing teems with dynamism and determination, driven toward visions of a better world for society and for nursing's place in achieving these greater social ends. Toward this goal, nursing strains to release its potential, to assert its values and capabilities, and to increase its voice and stature in the scheme of things. Regulation is central to this transformation. On the one hand it brings order to the movement, and on the other it provides social sanction for its objectives. (International Council of Nurses, 1986)

This statement is the key to this paper. It describes health care and nursing as dynamic forces and the need for nursing to develop and to release its potential for the public good. It also refers to the central and enabling role of regulation.

Five years earlier the World Health Organization published its report *Nursing in Support of the Goal Health for All by the Year 2000* (WHO, 1982). This report recorded that:

> Nursing practice and education are governed by legislation that is often archaic, determined by persons from other disciplines, detrimental to the status of the nurse, and not in tune with the needs of society. The primary health care strategy involves the re-evaluation of old policies and this must certainly include nursing legislation.

What, then, is the position in the UK and how do we withstand the criticism I have quoted? Such criticism would at least to some extent have been deserved if we were meeting before 1986. In that year the UKCC proposals for the reform of nursing education were published. Now accepted in principle by the government, these propose an entirely new basis for nursing education in the UK. They include a new emphasis on community care, in addition to 'institutional' care, greater flexibility, improved programmes of preparation and a new focus on health and its promotion. Perhaps, above all, the proposals are a recognition that the nursing professions are not currently prepared adequately to meet the present and future health needs of society. By definition, there is the profound implication that nursing is not attaining its potential to meet the real needs of the society the profession exists to serve. Project 2000 is part of the direct and future strategic answer to the words of Margretta Styles. What then are the impediments to progress?

The first impediment is the semantic problem, the fundamental misunderstandings that can hamper real progress. Words are often used without clear meaning and incorrect messages can be conveyed. What is often clear and well defined to the user of terms is often nothing of the sort to the recipient. Take three terms for example: practising nurse, practice nurse, nurse practitioner. These illustrate the scope for confusion.

Practising nurse in the UK is generally used to denote a nurse whose name appears on the professional register held by the UKCC. *Practice nurse*, on the other hand, has quite another meaning. This is used to denote a nurse employed by a GP of a medical practice. In this role, the practice nurse will undertake a range of clinical responsibilities which are not necessarily uniform and may differ in scope between practices. *Nurse practitioner* has a materially different connotation. It is used to denote a level of clinical activity and responsibility that goes beyond the 'conventional' role of nursing practitioners. Included in this may be the activity of limited diagnosis and prescription.

This discussion is now beginning to shift away from semantics to a much more fundamental question of professional practice and the scope and boundaries between professions.

The 1979 Nurses, Midwives and Health Visitors Act charges the UKCC with the responsibility not only to establish but also to improve standards of training and professional conduct. In governing nursing, midwifery and health visiting, the Council is involved in determining standards and developing strategies for its responsibilities to be fulfilled, often with the collaboration of the National Board for Nursing, Midwifery and Health Visiting in England, Northern Ireland, Scotland and Wales.

Subordinate legislation – set out in Statutory Instrument 1983 No.873 – embodies statements on the competence required of first and second level registered nurses. The Council is formally consulting on the proposed rules for the standard, kind and content of future pre-registration nursing education based on the Project 2000 proposals.

In addition to the legislation described, the Council has a code of professional conduct and has issued papers containing additional advice and elaboration of the Code. The Code is both a statement of the values of the profession and an explicit expression of the primacy of patients and clients. In the context of this paper, it is especially pertinent to say that the Code requires individual practitioners to exercise their discretion and judgement, at all times, in the interests of those in their care.

Just as nursing legislation exists, so, too, does legislation for medical practice, pharmaceutical and other areas of professional practice.

What, then, is the relevance of this legislative and regulatory position to the nurse practitioner concept as we loosely understand it? The legislation to which I have referred establishes boundaries of practice and ascribes discrete spheres and responsibilities to practitioners.

The development of any clinical nursing role cannot therefore be seen in isolation. The impact of extending the boundaries of nursing practice will often influence the boundaries of medical or other practice. Similarly, expansions in medical practice, or the negotiated delegation of some medical activities to nurses by doctors, will have an impact on the boundary of nursing practice. I have restricted my comments to legislative issues – but of course there are employment ones and others that emerge from policy developments and local initiatives. Within the UK the acceptance of so-called extended responsibilities has been addressed by the government health departments and others. A policy framework exists for how this could be negotiated and approached in the public health service. There is no obstacle to progress in this area, provided the commitment is there.

Issues to be addressed

If the concept of the nurse practitioner is to develop in a positive way, a number of issues must be addressed.

Let us recall that health care and nursing are dynamic forces. Doctors and nurses in clinical practice work closely and collaborate together. As trust and teamwork develops, usually based on the mutual recognition of the skills and complementary contribution of each to each in care, boundaries inevitably begin to change. These may not always be of a highly planned or formal kind but are more a consequence of the development of inter-professional trust and understanding and improved treatment and practice. New approaches to treatment have and will continue to alter and develop practice and lead, in the first instance, to an informal adjustment of boundaries. Gradually, tasks and responsibilities can shift from the practitioner of one profession to a practitioner of another.

Alternatively, and especially in some areas of community care, an unmet need may be perceived by a nurse and local initiatives taken to ensure that the need is met.

Circumstances such these are not uncommon and can develop to varying degrees. The effect on boundaries arises in the case of nursing, when a nurse strays into territory formerly bounded by medical practice. Alternatively, practice may develop in uncharted or unoccupied territory and the general principles that follow also apply to this situation.

There are a number of consequences and challenges. The first is that it can create an invidious position for the practitioner and two matters should be resolved before proceeding. Is the new element of the nursing role is a logical extension of the caring role of the nurse and of the scope of nursing practice, and, if this is accepted, will the 'primary' caring role be compromised? The second consequence is the personal liability of the practitioner in assuming a new aspect of practice, and indeed, if there is another professional involved, the personal liability of the practitioner who may have 'authorised' the assumption of new responsibilities.

The third consequence also concerns the individuals involved. If we consider the worst outcome of a clinical event, when harm may befall a patient or client, negligent delegation of responsibility by a doctor to a nurse is no mitigation for the acceptance of the responsibility by a nurse. Any nurse in such a position must first agree to accept responsibilities and is expected to meet the requirements of the UKCC Code of Conduct to which I have referred. Implicit in this requirement is that she is competent to accept them and that the interests of the patient and client are observed and protected.

A fourth consequence is that events and developments in clinical practice and care occur initially in the clinical setting. The result is that changes in practice take place before policies can be formulated by nursing and other managers and advisers. In addition, appropriate adjustments to the nursing educational curriculum usually follow, not precede, developments in practice. This is a fact of life in clinical practice. The sensitivity of professional managers, advisers and educators is required. It should equally be recognised that there is, inevitably and unavoidably, a phase between developments occuring and the position being 'formalised' in some way.

I do not draw attention to this for bureaucratic reasons; I stress this phase because it is during this period when clinical practice alters, and with it a changed shape in the boundary of the professions or professionals involved. This phase, which I would like to describe as the 'pioneering phase', is usually the most vulnerable for the patient, client and practitioner.

By definition, pioneers take risks. In clinical care, the risks must be highly calculated and may be designed to establish new frontiers. Above all they must safeguard and protect the position of consumers and recipients of care, who should be involved in their 'mapping' and 'planning' as far as possible.

I have discussed the proposed reforms of nursing education, the semantic problem, the framework for professional regulation and the position of practitioners when boundaries of practice change. I have also drawn attention to the challenge to those involved.

Professional regulation exists to safeguard standards in the public interest. It is not an impediment to progress or innovation – quite the reverse. Neither is regulation synonymous with restrictive practice. The regulatory process must be relevant and sensitive to changing health care and be able to alter and accommodate appropriate developments in practice.

The future

What then of the future? How should discussion of this concept proceed and in what context?

The reforms of pre-registration nursing education create a new opportunity to consider post registration education and concepts of specialist and advanced practice in nursing, midwifery and health visiting. The UKCC is reviewing this position and this may, at the very least, create a new chance to consider terminology and eliminate some of the scope for confusion.

The UKCC is also developing effective collaborative links with the General Medical Council to consider matters of mutual concern and develop greater understanding between our two professions. Collaboration of this kind should be mirrored at all levels of health care and is an essential ingredient if better understanding is to be achieved and the public is to be well and properly served.

In addition, a group representative of the medical, pharmaceutical and nursing professions has been convened by the Department of Health in England to consider nurse prescribing. I am pleased that the UKCC is represented on this group and hope that positive results will emerge. I also hope that inter-professional collaboration and understanding will be improved.

As an aside let me relate further some earlier work I came across when working on accountability in practice. In 1961, a Dutch professor of social medicine, Dr A. Querido, spoke at a European symposium on higher education in nursing. He said:

> If Napoleon had emphasized the military importance of nurses as he did doctors, if the Crimean War had been fought twenty years earlier, if Florence Nightingale had started her work in a civilian organisation instead of in an army, scientific nursing would probably have been firmly established in the hospital at the time the physician made it his workshop for research and teaching. Instead of being the servant girl to medicine, nursing would in that case have entered into an equal partnership with medical practice, serving the patient from different sources of knowledge and skill as Florence Nightingale hoped to achieve.
>
> (World Health Organization, 1972)

How rules and indeed cultures can change with time is indicated in clear terms by Thomstad, describing a nurse and doctor who worked out new rules for a doctor-nurse game during their collaboration as co-directors of a comprehensive child health centre (Thomstad, 1973). They discuss the difficulties, often painful, of developing new working relationships and the benefits that can be expected despite the high personal cost of negotiating the new rules. Let me give you three examples of their old and new rules:

1. Old rules say: 'Medical care is more important than nursing care.' New rules say: 'Good health care requires both good nursing care and good medical care.'
2. Old rules say: 'The doctor knows more than the nurse.' New rules say: 'Good doctors know more medicine than good nurses; good nurses know more nursing than good doctors.'
3. Old rules say: 'Good doctors rarely make mistakes and see to it that others don't either.' New rules say: 'Everyone makes mistakes, but open communication between doctors and nurses minimises them.'

I hope I have provided a general impression of the development of clinical roles within the regulatory context. In conclusion I would make three pleas, which are also my ingredients for a strategy.

The first is the need for extreme care in the use of titles and terms. I have talked earlier about the semantic problems we face; we already have an array of titles and terms which often bewilder consumers of health care, particularly nursing care. The focus should be on articulating the elements of the nurse practitioner role that are fundamentally different from those of existing nursing roles before the new role becomes a complete blueprint. A solution may be found in addressing the inadequacies of the current position rather than superimposing a new role which may only address the symptom of the problem, not the problem itself.

My second plea concerns the need to recognise the relationship between the proposed reforms in pre-registration nursing education and the forthcoming consideration by the UKCC of post-registration education and practice. The Project 2000 report referred to the notion of specialist practitioners and this should be the subject of further analyses and debate. What, for example, are the distinctions in the UK between practising in a speciality and being a specialist? What, too, of other clinical specialist roles that have been developed in areas other than primary care, including accident and emergency, rheumatology and the homeless? Is the exercise of clinical skill and judgement by a clinical specialist in oncology, a primary nurse, stoma care or AIDS nursing of a comparable order to those of nurse practitioners?

My third plea is to set all of these considerations in context. In the UK we anticipate demographic changes that will have considerable impact on staffing health services and recruitment.

We have reviews of the health services and increasing discussion on how these should or could be provided, and a debate about the appropriate lead agency role between some aspects of health and social services. There is a natural focus on cost-effectiveness and outcomes. We will see the development of a new support worker role for the care sector. This provides a new opportunity for nursing, midwifery and health visiting to examine critically the nature of support required to allow professional time to be applied where it is most needed – in the care of patients and clients. Not only will this lead to a change in skill and team mix, but it will also create new opportunities for those with ability and desire to progress. These opportunities are denied to many at the moment.

New directions and strategies can be determined, and consensus secured, by collaboration, co-operation and frank debate. Progress may be by a series of shuffles or by great leaps. What matters is that it **is** progress.

References

International Council of Nurses (1986), *The Regulation of Nursing* (based on a project report by Margretta Styles for

the Professional Services Committee of the International
Council of Nurses and accepted by the Council of National
Representatives, June 1985). Geneva: ICN.

Thomstad, B. *et al* (1973), 'Changing the rules of the
doctor-nurs

World Hea   n
Nursing: R   3
November 1   r
Europe.

World Heal   e
Goal Health

[handwritten note:]
Casey Hith Care Nurse —
Diploma ↑ P/Nursing
↓ ↓ Pathway
ambiguous + misleading
+ we're all —
practitioners
↓ Novice — skills

12 The role of professional organisations

TREVOR CLAY

In this paper I shall discuss the role of professional organisations in supporting the primary health care nurse, in the context of the growing debate about the role of the nurse practitioner and her niche in British primary health care.

I shall refer throughout my paper to the role of professional trade unions. This is not intended to be a pedantic distinction: for example, the Royal College of Nursing has a dual function, and both functions are indispensable to the development of the nurse practitioner. As a professional body and royal college incorporated by charter, the RCN is concerned to advance the art and science of nursing. It carries the responsibility for protecting safe practice and promoting its development. As a trade union, it must protect and indemnify its members. It carries the representative authority and negotiating strength to secure the changes it desires.

The RCN supports the development of the nurse practitioner role in British primary health care. It believes that the nurse practitioner can meet an existing and urgent consumer need, and is committed to promoting the legislative and organisational changes needed to translate the pioneering work of individual innovators into living reality. Our support for the nurse practitioner is founded in our analysis of historical developments in health provision, likely future trends and confidence in the capacity of nurses to extend their skilled contribution within the primary health care team.

The major improvements in the health status of the British population have been achieved this century primarily through public health measures such as slum clearance, Clean Air Acts and the construction of sewers. All nurses and medical practitioners should remember this salient fact. These measures were followed by qualitative leaps forward in medical science and technology in the middle years of the century. I believe we have now reached a plateau in medical technology and science, from which it will be very difficult to launch another great leap forward. Most commentators are agreed that major qualitative advance can now be expected principally from improving the infrastructure and delivery of primary health care, particularly preventative care and health promotion. These are mass systems of health delivery. Medicine does not have the manpower: nursing has both the numbers and the skill.

The RCN therefore supports the philosophy behind the 1987 government White Paper on primary health care, and was pleased to note that additional funds for primary health care services were earmarked. A pity, then, that the government has chosen the wrong mechanism for implementing its strategy: a strategy that relies almost exclusively on family practitioner committees and cash incentives for general practitioners is fatally flawed.

Success in the field of health promotion depends on modifying the behaviour of the individual. The nurse is particularly well equipped for this role. If we are serious about achieving health promotion objectives, then all health care professionals must make a balanced assessment, in the interests of the consumer, of the practitioner most likely to achieve success. Our aim must be to empower the consumer – to help clients and patients to take control of their own destiny and understand their own health needs.

Doctor consultation time remains severely limited, their counselling skills are not necessarily highly developed and their training and ethos is still essentially disease-focused and curative. I will not rehearse the clear evidence that nurses are acceptable to the consumer and achieve a better rapport with clients and better take-up of health advice and treatment than doctors.

One further point on choosing the right professional for the task – surely only a mass profession like nursing can hope to rise to the challenge of mass screening, advice and education.

Empowering the nurse

I have talked of the need to empower the consumer. We also have to empower the nurse, and here the professional trade union has a crucial role. The nurse must be indemnified for her practice and must be accountable for her practice. Indeed the accountability comes first: it is the essential pre-requisite for an extension of the nurse's role. The nurse must, through appropriate basic and post-basic education, recognise the limits of her own competence and be accountable for her practice.

Without the professional indemnity given to nurse practitioners Barbara Stilwell and Barbara Burke-Masters, their pioneering work could have been seriously hampered. They are secure in their professionalism and skill base, but on other occasions the RCN has had to sound a note of warning to groups – including some practice nurses – not to be over-confident of their competence. And while the RCN supported Barbara Burke-Masters, it does not subscribe to the view that nurse practitioners are simply there to fill gaps in unpopular areas of practice left by GPs, as was the case with the homeless in London.

The nurse's code of professional conduct must be defined sufficiently widely to allow her to work as a nurse practitioner. The RCN will work with the UKCC to establish the right framework and will indemnify appropriately trained professionals.

The creation of the right framework begins with nurses' basic education. The Project 2000 reforms are essential if the employment of nurse practitioners is to take off. The new curricula will, we hope, produce a flexible, assertive professional, equipped to work in both hospital and community. The RCN has played a key role in promoting the reform of nurse education and will now argue for recognition of postbasic qualifications identifying competence as a nurse practitioner. In many parts of the country the nurse practitioner is clearly an extension of the district nurse or health visitor role. We will build on what we have, rather than create a new animal from scratch. The RCN has already drawn on the expertise of leading professionals to develop a training programme for the nurse practitioner through its Institute of Advanced Nursing Education. Ultimately, it will be necessary to seek to influence the national boards to recognise, develop and accredit appropriate postbasic courses.

To recapitulate the necessary ingredients for securing a clear niche for the nurse practitioner in British primary health care, we need the support of the profession and its statutory body, we need appropriately trained and indemnified professionals, and we need to promote consensus within the health care team that nurses are the appropriate professionals to meet the primary health care challenge.

To promote that consensus, we need more research into why nurse practitioners are successful. Research has already demonstrated that the nurse practitioner can be acceptable to the consumer, is competent in diagnosis, does not miss problems and refers appropriately to other health professionals. It also indicates that nurses achieve better take-up or compliance with health advice than doctors do. Clients too demonstrate quite a sophisticated understanding of those conditions and problems which will be appropriately dealt with by the nurse practitioner. However, not enough is known about the reasons underlying this. The RCN will fight nursing's corner in the battle to improve the paltry resources available to nursing research – paltry, that is, when weighed against the £450 million a year devoted to medical research – but do not construe my plea for qualitative research and follow-up as an argument for delay. We need the nurse practitioner and we need her now because we are failing to meet consumer need.

When we look to create the right framework for the nurse practitioner, it is important that we recognise where she already exists. Although current interest focuses on the nurse working in the GP clinic or health centre, the RCN is firm about placing this development in the wider context of primary care. There are already many nurse practitioners at work. They may be disguised as occupational health nurses; as midwives – particularly independent midwives; they may be found in some accident and emergency departments; and there are many specialists in rheumatology, diabetes, stoma care and terminal or palliative care who fit the RCN's concept of a nurse practitioner.

Other nurses display elements of the nurse practitioner role, or have clear potential for developing in this direction. They include district nurses, who are currently constrained by health authority hierarchies which limit their control over their caseload and by their lack of prescribing powers. Health visitors are perhaps too over burdened with responsibilities for children under five for their potential to take off, and of course many specialist nurses are constrained in the same way as district nurses by their lack of authority to prescribe.

Practice nurses and treatment room nurses are obvious candidates for training as nurse practitioners but we will need to secure the necessary training programmes. Practice nurses have been flavour of the month with the Department of Health; its plans for women's health, involving clinic or health-centre based screening, could generate a key role for practice nurses. They are of course employed by GPs, on whom the Department's primary health care strategy relies.

However, the emergence of practice nurses as nurse practitioners could well serve as a symbol for the opportunities and dilemmas facing the profession. Should the profession and the college take a pragmatic line and simply accept delegated authority for the nurse from the GP, with the GP as the principal assessor of the practice nurse's competence? It would be relatively easy then to win GPs' acceptance of the nurse practitioner role. But, and it is a big but, should we not instead assert our professional autonomy and conduct our discussions and negotiations at a more formal level, between representative bodies, especially as so many practice nurses lack community training?

Professional autonomy and the nurse's professional image are closely linked. It will be difficult for the concept of the nurse practitioner to gain acceptance if stereotypical attitudes to nursing persist. As the dominant voice in nursing, the RCN has to take on the work of combatting the traditional image of nurses. After all, the angel model encapsulates all the barriers towards progress in primary health care and for the nurse practitioner. It reinforces the notion of the nurse as handmaiden to the doctor. It asserts the dominance of the medical model and of the hospital sector and it carries the implication that nurses are caring ... but not terribly bright!

In this context, it is important that professional trade unions like the RCN both inform and reassure colleagues from other health disciplines by highlighting the fact that nurse practitioners already exist. Indeed groups like occupational health nurses and midwives already have a legislative framework which could be adapted to extend prescribing powers to nurse practitioners. It may require a revolution in attitudes, but it only needs an evolution in existing regulations to achieve change.

Individual nurses cannot hope to translate their aspirations for professional development into practice without the active support of their professional trade union. To achieve change, whether evolutionary or revolutionary, representative authority and political clout is needed. As an example, the RCN's active participation in the primary health care roadshows associated with the Cumberlege review, and its espousal of the Cumberlege recommendations, have been crucially important in gaining their professional and political acceptance.

Since the Cumberlege review and the publication of the 1987 White Paper, the RCN has been engaged in continuing dialogue with the medical and pharmaceutical professions to promote acceptance of nurse prescribing and develop practical protocols for its implementation. Considerable progress has been made in this area, with the acceptance by the British Medical Association and the General Medical Services Committee of the principle of nurse prescribing. In Parliament, the RCN will continue to seek opportunities to amend the 1968 Medicines Act as part of its wider lobbying to improve MPs' understanding of nurses' existing skills and the potential of the nurse practitioner. The profession is treading a careful path – keen to achieve a consensus of support among the medical and pharmaceutical professions, but determined also to assert nurses' professional autonomy.

At the heart of the RCN's support for the nurse practitioner is a commitment to empowering the consumer and to consumer choice. This commitment forms the central plank of its strategy for maintaining and developing the NHS. In the recently published report of the Royal College of Nursing's independent commission on the NHS (RCN 1988), It is argued that people should have the right of direct access to a variety of health practitioners, including those offering complementary therapies. This report was submitted as evidence to the Prime Minister's review of the NHS, and its recommendations will be promoted in the continuing public and parliamentary debate on future patterns of health care delivery.

A secure place for the nurse practitioner in British primary health care would give practical expression to the ideal of greater choice, education and responsibility for consumers. The RCN is committed to achieving that ideal.

Reference

Royal College of Nursing (1988), *The Health Challenge*, London: RCN.

13 Power and policy-making in nursing

JANE ROBINSON

'Skill mix' is today's buzz phrase. Gray (1988) offers two economic definitions: the proportional composition of the nursing labour force by grade, and the distribution of tasks by grade of nurse (other worker). I have invented a definition of my own derived perhaps from conspiracy theory – 'skill mix: a coded term used to conceal the deliberate substitute of a lower grade (educated/paid) worker for a higher grade (educated/paid) worker in order to carry out the same tasks for lower cost'.

Feminist authors Phillips and Taylor (1980) offer another related definition:

> Skill definitions are saturated with sexual bias. The work of women is often deemed inferior simply because it is women who do it. Women workers carry into the workplace their status as subordinate individuals, and this status comes to define the value of the work they do. Far from being an objective economic fact, skill is often an ideological category imposed on certain types of work by virtue of the sex and power of the workers who perform it. (p. 216)

From their point of view questions of skill mix, or the division of labour, are to do with status and power. I agree. In *New Model Management: Griffiths and the NHS* (Strong and Robinson, 1988) we suggested that status in the NHS can be conceptualised very simply – doctors at the top, everyone else underneath:

The NHS is merely a system for servicing individual doctors. As such, its essential structure is that of a pyramid. At its apex stands a relatively tiny group of individual doctors (with consultants perhaps a little higher than general practitioners). Each has to cope with the sometimes grave responsibility of managing disease but each has also been trained in the best of modern scientific medicine.

Below them, stretching out in ever vaster numbers towards the base of the pyramid, come the support staff; those who nurture, aid and facilitate the work of each doctor – around a million in total. Put crudely, on one side stand the subordinate men: engineers, porters, adminstrators, ambulancemen, groundsmen, accountants, electricians, psychiatric nurses and scientists without medical degrees. On the other side are the subordinate women: general nurses, cleaners, clerks, social workers, health visitors, laboratory technicians, the 'professions ancillary to medicine'. But, though the jobs and genders are often different, they are handmaidens all. (p. 55-6)

To put the matter in a nutshell, these are the social relationships within which work in the NHS is embedded. It is not the nature of the tasks which is as important as the social context in which they are carried out (Pahl, 1988). It is a context firmly rooted in a particular, historical distribution of power. Any attempt to extend or expand traditional roles means not just negotiating for space at the margins of the divisions of labour, but also challenging a status quo in which one occupational group – the doctors – have long since staked out the territory.

I have a model (not, I hasten to add, a nursing model!) which seems to have caught people's imagination when demonstrating how I see the nurses' case in the division of labour. It came to me when I was asked to be

Figure 2   The Nurses' House

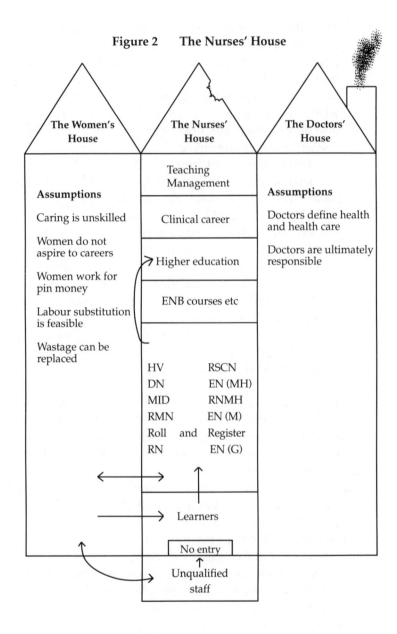

'constructive' in a paper on the nursing labour crisis. In the light of the evidence I found it very hard to be constructive, but the word suggested building something – a construction which (like the tower blocks of the 1960s) could be built, but then, if unpopular or inappropriate, could be demolished. So I came upon the idea of constructing a nurses' house (Figure 2).

What, I asked myself, would such a house look like? Very tall and thin, I thought, and really rather dilapidated. The house has few windows because the people on the inside rarely look out, and its roof is sorely in need of repair. This nurses' house is positively squashed between a very big house on one side, and a very posh one on the other. The huge house is the women's house, and it is so large that it contains more than half the people in the world. The posh house belongs to the doctors – and it's a very grand affair with a brass knocker, a chimney and a beautiful garden.

Almost all of the people who live in the nurses' house come in from the women's house, and on that side it has three doors. On the doctor's side it has only a peephole. One door goes down the steps from the garden on the women's side into the cellar. The women who go in there have big labels on their aprons saying 'unqualified', but once in the cellar they all work terribly hard and do almost the same jobs as the nurses upstairs. But on the inside of the house the door to the cellar is locked and bolted, and if any of the women want to move upstairs they have to go out through the garden again, and into the second door marked 'learners'.

The learners' door is very big because so many people keep going in and out. Indeed, if you stop and count them you will find that for every three learners that go in, one comes out. The learners, too, work terribly hard and seem to do most of the housework. If they put up with the work they stay in that part of the house for three years, and then they are called 'qualified' and allowed upstairs.

The upstairs part of the house is very odd. It has lots of rooms which qualified nurses live in with the doors tightly shut. They hardly ever go outside their rooms, which have notices on the doors saying things like RMN or RGN or Enrolled Nurse, Mental Handicap. It is very peculiar, because the rooms all look the same inside – except for different patterned wallpaper or perhaps an unusual lampshade.

Sometimes the qualified nurses get pretty bored and try to think of ways to make their lives more interesting. A few go and spend two or three years in other rooms, and as a result many of them have collected lots of the different door notices. Some can show you piles with RMN, RM, RHV, DN, RSCN as well as RGN on them. But they still seem to go on doing the same jobs.

Some of the bored nurses think there is no reason why they should not take on some of the jobs from the chaps next door in the doctors' house. More often than not, after peeping through the spyhole, the nurses notice that the chaps do not do many of their jobs anyway – and those that do are pretty incompetent (things like listening to people). So these enterprising nurses put forward plans to help the chaps, pointing out how frightfully busy they always are, and how much cheaper it would be to use a nurse. But as soon as the doctors hear about this they start shouting back through the hole in the wall. 'You can't do that', they bellow, 'it's illegal, it's our job, keep off.'

So about half of these qualified nurses get fed up and leave the house by the third door marked 'escape route' – they get married and have babies, and even run employment agencies for nurses. Just a few stay in the nurses' house and try to get over their boredom by going up the nursing hierarchy, which means climbing the stairs to the attic. Even fewer try to go up on the outside via the higher education fire escape. But they have to keep dashing back in order to do the work and some of them fall off the ladder – or just get so tired they give up.

The nurses' house has looked like this for almost a hundred years. Every so often the landlord brings them a tin of sweets and the nurses are always grateful. Once they have eaten them they keep the tins to show on the mantelpiece – there's one with a label 'Nurses' Act 1919', and another 'Briggs Committee', and yet another just called 'Halsbury'. Currently they are trying the sweets from a tin labelled 'Project 2000', although some of the nurses are not sure whether the toffees really agree with them.

So what will happen to the nurses' house in the next hundred years? Given that the main feature of any status quo is a huge resistance to change, my guess would be – not a great deal. Concessions may appear to be given, but when the dust has cleared everything remains the same. Caring is believed to be unskilled women's work; women are assumed to work for pin money and not for careers, and the papers we have heard do not reassure me that the role of the nurse practitioner would bring about a sea change. The case for the role seemed to be argued in two parts (Table 1).

Proponents of the status quo can simply take those aspects of the role that are useful to their ends. If technical skills are in short supply then they will be appropriately rewarded and the status of the associated jobs will rise. The skills of 'women's work', on the other hand, are invariably assumed to be ubiquitous – there is little status to be gained in the world of work from being an empathetic listener and teacher, or mistress of the 'dirty work'.

The projected shortage of appropriately qualified school leavers has given rise to a flurry of activity in nurse recruitment (and may, more than anything else, have assured the government's acceptance of Project 2000). Yet, on the other side of the coin, more and more women are entering the labour market – an estimated 1 million between 1986 and 1995 (Institute for Employment

Research, 1987). And as medicine moves gradually to having a 50 per cent female membership, some rearrangement of the internal division of labour will be needed there. Sex discrimination at work is another powerfully entrenched phenomenon and it does not take too great a leap of the imagination to envisage all those part-time women doctors carrying out, in the year 2010, the very tasks that the nurse practitioner lays claim to in 1988.

So is the future of the extended development of nursing all doom and gloom? Paradoxically I see a way forward, not through professionalising strategies, but through common sense alliances. The writing of the academic sociologist of medicine, Freidson, can be taken as a marker for recent attitudinal changes towards the professions. In 1973 he was writing about society's increasing dependence on specialised knowledge and skill; by 1986 he was describing how the management of medicine has come to represent the most serious challenge to its organisation and political strength. The irony of the professionalising strategy is that nursing has missed the boat. We know now that claims to certain privileges in the name of a public service ethic have led too often to narrow, self-serving monopolies of interest. Ironically, it has often been the adherents to trade unionism rather than the professionals who have identified most with patient or client concerns, despite their reputed preoccupation with members' interests over public good.

Some nurses were most offended when we suggested in *New Model Management* that the way forward is through regarding nursing as an honest trade. Yet nurses' challenge to the status quo could come about by focusing on the institution and its goals rather than on enhancing nursing's power. Standards of performance have to be set, and the consumer's voice and choice should assume a far greater place on the agenda. Indeed it is through a far greater sense of partnership with the inhabitants of the women's house (as well as the doctors' house) that I see a way forward. Such an approach could force a debate on questions of the effectiveness, efficiency, equity and humanity of health care systems. It is in this arena that nurses could play a greater part. The extended role of the nurse may indeed prove to be most cost-effective in certain situations (although such proof is fraught with difficulty Marks 1985) but that alone is not enough. We also have to ask whether such a role promotes the more equitable and humane delivery of health care. Answering that question might involve a mighty spring clean in the nurses' house. Making friends with the neighbours on both sides of the fence could mean that the house in the middle took on a whole new look.

References

Freidson, E. (ed) (1973), *The Professions and their Prospects*, New York: Sage.

Freidson, E. (1986), *Professional Powers: a study of the institutionalisation of formal knowledge*, Chicago: University of Chicago Press.

Gray, A. (1988), 'What cost skill mix?' Paper delivered to the Manpower Society, November 17.

Institute for Employment Research, (1987), *Review of the Economy and Employment*. Institute for Employment Research, University of Warwick.

Marks, I. (1985), *Psychiatric Nurse Therapists in Primary Care: the expansion of advanced clinical roles in nursing*, London: Royal College of Nursing.

Pahl, R. (ed) (1988), *On Work: Historical, comparative and theoretical approaches*, Oxford: Basil Blackwell.

Phillips, A. and Taylor, B. (1980), 'Sex and skill: notes towards a feminist economics', *Feminist Review*, 6,79, quoted in Evans, J. (ed) (1982), *The Woman Question: readings in the subordination of women*, Oxford: Fontana.

Strong, P. and Robinson, J. (1988), *New model management: Griffiths and the NHS*, Nursing Policy Studies Centre, University of Warwick.

Key references

These references appear frequently throughout this publication, so for brevity they are cited in full only once, in this list.

Department of Health and Social Security (1986), *Neighbourhood Nursing: A focus for care* (the Cumberlege report), London: HMSO.

Department of Health and Social Security (1986), *Primary Health Care: An agenda for discussion*, London: HMSO.

Department of Health and Social Security (1987), *Promoting Better Health: The government's programme for improving primary health*, London: HMSO.

Department of Health and Social Security (1988), *Public Health in England* (the Acheson report), London: HMSO.

Griffiths, R. (1988), *Community Care: Agenda for action*, London: HMSO.

UK Central Council for Nursing, Midwifery and Health Visiting (1986), *Project 2000: A new preparation for practice*, London: UKCC.

UK Central Council for Nursing, Midwifery and Health Visiting (1984), *Code of Professional Conduct*, London: UKCC.

World Health Organization (1985), *Targets for Health for All by the Year 2000*, Copenhagen: WHO Regional Office for Europe.

Appendix: Seminar participants

This list includes participants who attended by invitation part or all of the seminar and follow-up day, with the posts they occupied at that time. They were taking part as individuals, not as delegates representing the views of their organisations or employers.

Ms Virginia Beardshaw	Policy Analyst, King's Fund Institute, UK.
Professor Nicholas Bosanquet	Professor of Health Policy, Royal Holloway and Bedford New College, Universityof London, UK.
Ms Pearl Brown	Assistant Unit General Manager, Islington Health Authority, UK.
Professor Tony Butterworth	Queen's Nursing Institute Professor of Community Nursing, University of Manchester, UK.
Dr John Chisholm	Chairman, Practice Organisation Sub-Committee, British Medical Association; general practitioner, UK.
Dr June Clark	Chief Nursing Adviser, Harrow Health Authority, UK.

Mrs Julia Cumberlege	Chairman, South West Thames Regional Health Authority, UK.
Mrs Anne Dant	Practice Nurse, Cleveland, UK.
Mrs Ami David	Primary Health Care Group, King's Fund Centre, UK.
Ms Denise Dennehy	Nursing Officer (International Relations), Department of Health, UK.
Dr Mary O'Hara Devereaux	Director, Planning and Education, Hawaii University, USA.
Mr William Doughty	Chairman, North West Thames Regional Health Authority, UK.
Dr Marie Farrell	Regional Officer for Nursing, Midwifery and Social Work Services, World Health Organisation Regional Office for Europe.
Mrs Ainna Fawcett-Henesy	Chief Nursing Adviser, Ealing Health Authority, UK.

Miss Elaine Fullard

Project Director, Oxford Prevention of Heart Attack and Stroke Project, UK.

Ms Shirley Goodwin

General Secretary, Health Visitors Association, UK.

Miss Margaret Green

Director of Education, Royal College of Nursing, UK.

Miss Doreen Horridge

Nursing Officer, Department of Health, UK.

Mr Chris Kenny

Principal, Community Services Division, Department of Health, UK.

Dr Ronald King

Regional Postgraduate Dean, South East Thames Regional Health Authority, UK.

Dr Amelia Mangay Maglacas

Chief Scientist for Nursing, World Health Organization.

Dr Robert Maxwell

Secretary, King Edward's Hospital Fund for London, UK.

Ms Evelyn McEwen

Divisional Director of
Services, Age Concern, UK.

Mrs Makhwade

Chief Nurse/Assistant Director
of Hospital Services, Botswana.

Mr Colin Ralph

Registrar and Chief Executive,
UK Central Council for Nursing,
Midwifery and Health Visiting.

Dr Geoffrey Rivett

Senior Principal Medical Officer,
Department of Health, UK.

Dr Jane Robinson

Director, Nursing Policy Studies
Centre, University of Warwick,
UK.

Mrs Barbara Robottom

Professional Adviser
(District Nursing),
English National Board for
Nursing, Midwifery and Health
Visiting, UK.

Ms Jane Salvage

Director,
Nursing Developments,
King's Fund Centre, UK.

Dr Theo Schofield

Lecturer in general practice,
University of Oxford;
general practitioner,
Warwickshire, UK.

Ms Barbara Stilwell

Nurse practitioner
and researcher, UK.

Ms Barbara Stocking

Director,
King's Fund Centre,
UK.

Professor Jenifer Wilson-Barnett

Department of
Nursing, King's
College London,
UK.